THE BEVERLY HILLS

HILLS

Shape™

THE BEVERLY HILLS
HILLS
Shape
THE *TRUTH* ABOUT PLASTIC SURGERY

™

DR. STUART A. LINDER
Beverly Hills Plastic Surgeon

TAG

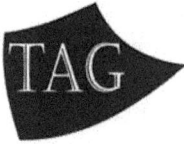

Quantity discounts are available on bulk orders.
Contact sales@TAGPublishers.com for more information.

TAG Publishing, LLC
2618 S. Lipscomb
Amarillo, TX 79109
www.TAGPublishers.com

Office (806) 373-0114
Fax (806) 373-4004
info@TAGPublishers.com

ISBN: 978-1-59930-316-1

First Edition

Dedication

This book is dedicated to the women and men throughout the world who desire to be educated in and informed of the best possible plastic surgery techniques of the body. My goal is to assist women and men in making fully informed and educated decisions when considering the life-changing experience that will occur with the sculpting of the body.

ACKNOWLEDGMENTS

It is with great honor and privilege that I have the opportunity to improve and enhance the self-image of people every day. Performing surgery, a perfect chain of brilliant people must come together to create the final outcome. I wish to extend my sincerest thanks and personal regard to all of those who have helped me to create this book for the betterment of those who are considering plastic surgery of the body.

I would first like to thank Crystal, my wife, for her constant companionship, wisdom, intelligence, and brilliance. It was with her encouragement and support that this project came into being. The need for the public to understand the qualifications of and safety in plastic surgery, and to be educated in the process, has always been my utmost concern. This book was created as a handbook to help educate and safeguard individuals who are considering elective surgery procedures.

Next, I thank my beautiful children, Blake and Alexis, who are the joy of my life. Watching them grow each and every day brings constant happiness and inspiration to my wife and I.

I thank my parents, who have raised six children to be professional, honorable, and ethical people who help those around them at all times.

I would like to take the opportunity to thank my surgical operating room team, including our anesthesiologist, who has performed thousands of general anesthetics for me with my patients over the years, with the highest of professional care at all times. Without excellent anesthesia, the results of plastic surgery can be devastating and/or disastrous.

I would like to thank our surgical technicians and nurses who work tirelessly, taking care of the patients both before surgery and in recovery, comforting them, and making their overall experience pleasant and comfortable.

I would like to thank all of my teachers and professors starting from medical school at the University of California, Los Angeles through my residency in general surgery and plastic surgical training. Without their teachings of operative skills and judgment, as well as their experience in performing plastic surgical procedures, I could never be the doctor that I am today.

I thank the American Board of Plastic Surgery and the American Society of Plastic Surgeons, who have created a system to produce outstanding, ethical, well-qualified and -trained plastic surgeons in which the public can be completely assured of the highest and utmost professionalism and the highest quality-care standard at all times.

Finally, I would like to give my thanks to Kandi Miller with LifeSuccess Publishing. She has worked tirelessly to create this book and make it as readable as possible for the public whom it is designed to help.

CONTENTS

INTRODUCTION

"I love Los Angeles. I love Hollywood. They're beautiful.
Everybody's plastic, but I love plastic. I want to be plastic."

– Andy Warhol

There's no question that today's society has an absolute obsession with beauty and body makeovers. From the time of the pharaohs in ancient Egypt to present-day Hollywood, things haven't changed much. People want to be beautiful, they want to feel better about themselves and they want perfection. As the population is spurred on by the media and by television shows, cosmetic procedures have increased dramatically over the last five years.

According to the statistics of the American Society of Plastic Surgeons, more than 10.2 million cosmetic surgery procedures were performed in 2005. The five most common cosmetic procedures were liposuction, then nose reshaping, followed by breast enhancement surgery, eyelid surgery, and tummy tuck. Over 324,000 liposuction procedures; 291,000 breast augmentations; and 135,000 tummy tucks were performed in 2005 within the United States of America. It is obvious that the way in which women and men perceive their bodies is a universal concern. Hollywood exponentially influences women's desire to enhance their breasts and sculpt their bodies, and this desire is found throughout the United States, extending from Rodeo Drive in California to Park Avenue in New York and from Detroit, Michigan, down to Dallas, Texas.

One of the most important decisions that you will ever make may be to undergo a cosmetic surgery procedure. Once you have elected to proceed, your body, hopefully, will be changed for the better and your self-image greatly improved. On the other hand, if you do not take proper measures to seek a qualified plastic surgeon, you may be left with irreparable and disastrous results. The patient must understand that having cosmetic surgery is in no way like buying a new pair of designer shoes or a brand-new luxury automobile. If you buy one of those products and it is defective, you can usually return it and get your money back. This is not so with cosmetic surgery. If you have horrible damage done to your body, this damage may be irreversible, and unfortunately, it cannot be returned.

The pros and cons of media exposure to cosmetic surgery should be noted as well. Every day television programs air on local television channels as well as on cable stations detailing plastic surgical procedures. The positive programs are the documentary specials such as those seen on the Discovery Health Channel. These specials give a tremendous educational advantage to the patient hoping to undergo a cosmetic surgery procedure. Presented in documentary format, the episodes show patients as they appear before their surgery explaining the specific desires they wish to satisfy through cosmetic surgery. Patients are then followed into the operating room, while the viewer hears descriptive narratives by well-qualified surgeons describing the procedures and showing the final postoperative results. New techniques can also be described on these educational shows; all this may help aid the patient in finding qualified plastic surgeons.

Unfortunately, the media's message can be detrimental as well. There are some programs that are not educational or documentary, which portray cosmetic procedures to be as quick and simple as getting your hair or nails done. Cosmetic surgery is a major surgical procedure that has risks and the potential for complications. Many of these surgeries are complex and require extended recovery time, but one does not often see this on television shows. The potential for harm is glossed over, an enormous disservice to the public and to the potential patient.

Performing multiple surgeries on the body at one time can also lead to devastating and potentially life-threatening outcomes. It is vital that the patient understands that the time restraints within the operating room, associated with anesthesia and possible blood loss, are in place for their protection and are an absolute necessity when undergoing cosmetic surgery. Any surgeon willing to push these boundaries for a standard procedure should be thoroughly questioned by the patient.

One alarming trend on some television shows is the use of incompetent surgeons who have no qualifications to perform the surgeries that they are describing. They frequently ignore accepted standards, such as adequately following up with the patient after surgery, to the patient's detriment. Always remember, a doctor's appearance on a television program does not imply that he or she is qualified to operate on you. You still must check credentials.

The Internet has also opened an enormous avenue for information regarding cosmetic surgery procedures, but the same precautions as those given for television programs apply. Do your homework. Anyone can have a great website these days, but you want only qualified physicians operating on you.

> "IF IT SOUNDS TOO GOOD TO BE TRUE THEN IT PROBABLY IS."

One precaution to keep in mind is that many patients are confronted with lowball prices for some plastic surgery procedures. Surgery normally requires general anesthesia; therefore, a board-certified anesthesiologist always should be present. Furthermore, the operating room should be Medicare state licensed or be a Quad A–certified facility. There should be standard staff, including surgical technicians, circulating nurses, and recovery room nurses. All of this costs the patient money, real money. So any super-low prices seen in newspaper ads, at the back of telephone books or on signs at bus stops should lead the patient to great cautiousness.

You should also be aware that there are only two FDA-approved breast implants available in the United States. They are produced by Inamed Corporation and Mentor Corporation. There are no inexpensively priced implants available in the United States.

If the price of the operation is at a level that seems too low for a certain geographical area, you must be extra careful and fully aware as to what you are going to receive. Sure, there is a possibility you will get satisfactory results, but there's a much greater possibility that you won't. Be careful, and remember the old saying: **"If it sounds too good to be true then it probably is."**

This book is designed to help educate both men and women on important details to keep in mind when considering a body sculpting procedure. The two main themes are the female form and how it changes over time, and how to find a qualified surgeon.

Concerning the female form, I will discuss how a woman's body changes from the teenage years to middle age, then to post-breast-feeding and post-lactation status. Advancing age and the issues involving increased skin laxity and fat deposits will also be explained. I will then discuss how massive weight loss affects the body and what you can do about it.

If you, the patient, take away a good understanding of the two basic elements discussed herein, I will have succeeded with my message of optimism and increased awareness for those considering a body sculpting procedure.

– Dr. Linder

CHAPTER 1
Where Do I Start?

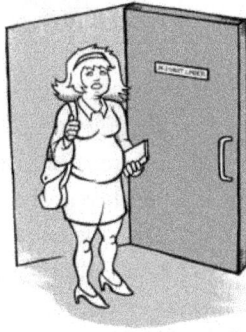

*"Even beauties can be unattractive. If you catch a beauty in
the wrong light at the right time . . . I believe in low lights
and trick mirrors. I believe in plastic surgery."*

– Andy Warhol

Hello, I'm Dr. Stuart Linder, and I am here to guide you through
the decision-making process as you consider some of the most
common body-sculpting procedures. I regard this opportunity as
quite a privilege. My goals are to educate you on the most popular
procedures available and then help you find the most qualified and
experienced surgeon to give you the best results possible.

First, let me tell you a little bit about myself. I have trained for
over thirteen years to become a plastic surgeon. That may seem like
a long time, but actually the time went quickly. I graduated medical
school from the UCLA School of Medicine, performed my residency
in general surgery, and then completed my fellowship in Plastic and

Reconstructive Surgery. I am board certified with the American Board of Plastic Surgery and am a member of the prestigious American Society of Plastic Surgeons. I have trained and am qualified in every aspect of plastic and reconstructive surgery, including cosmetic facial plastic surgery; but, with time, I have found my true passion. I deal with the body and the sculpting of the body to create normalcy, especially in correcting deformities, including congenital defects. As a result, I have completely dedicated my practice to the area of body sculpting.

WE HAVE ALSO PARTICIPATED IN MULTIPLE DOCUMENTARIES ON DISCOVERY HEALTH CHANNEL

My staff and I have performed thousands of body sculpting procedures and continue to perform hundreds of breast augmentations and reductions each year. I enjoy participating in documentaries for television because I feel it truly helps the patient by allowing them to watch these operations and see the beforeand-after results. We have worked with CBS News, NBC, Fox News, KTLA Los Angeles, K-Cal 9, Extra, MTV, E Channel, and the E! Hollywood Network. We have also participated in multiple documentaries on Discovery Health Channel, including specials such as "Breast Reduction," "Breast Augmentation," "Mommy Makeover," "Gigantomastic Breasts," "Body and Soul," "Correcting Breast Asymmetries," "Tubular Breast Deformity," "Abdominoplasty versus Liposuction" (on the Berman and Berman Show), "Breast Augmentation with Treacher Collins Syndrome," "Silicone Gel Implant Revision," and "Severe Congenital Breast Asymmetry." We have also worked with the Women's Entertainment Network (WE) on the Latin Breast Augmentation, The Learning Channel (TLC), NBC's The Other Half, Dick Clark Productions, and international television including CBS Germany, "Beverly Hills Body Sculpting," New Zealand Television Documentary for the American Music Awards, Azteca America, International Latin Television on "Breast Augmentation" and many, many more. Throughout all of these programs, the common thread is documenting safe and predictable surgery.

One major concern that I have these days is the number of patients that come to my practice each week requesting revision surgeries. Patients, especially in the Los Angeles area, are seen in my office almost daily with all types of severe breast deformities that are the aftermath of improperly performed breast augmentations, performed by non-board-certified surgeons. These doctors include physicians who are gynecologists, general surgeons, emergency room physicians, etc., and they are performing breast enhancements, tummy tucks and liposuctions with horrendous results. It is important to remember that any doctor in the state of California with a medical license can perform cosmetic surgery and that the consumer is unfortunately not in any way safeguarded from these physicians. This is the main reason I am writing this book: so that women and men can seek a qualified physician. It is my goal that this book will give you the information you need to make an intelligent choice.

There are patients who come into my office for breast implant revisions, but the damage is irreparable. They will never look normal, and I am saddened to tell them that I am unable to fix their breasts completely and make them look normal once again. I don't want this to happen to you; therefore, I have created a road map to help you understand the right questions to ask when considering any cosmetic procedure.

This book will cover several areas of body sculpting. The first area we will talk about is your own decision-making process. Why do you want to have surgery, and is it really what **you** want to do? I see women and men come into my office every week with unrealistic expectations. They expect to be magically transformed into a new person. You must understand that plastic surgery can only do so much, and while you can't look exactly the same as you did twenty-five years ago, you can still make meaningful improvements.

I have already briefly discussed the need to find a qualified and board-certified surgeon to perform your procedure. This is so important that I have dedicated a full chapter to the subject. I will tell you what questions you should ask and what answers you should be getting. Above all, I will encourage you to be very selective and thorough. This is your body, and the changes you are making can and will affect the rest of your life. Those changes can be very good if you do your homework, or they can be devastating and disfiguring if you don't.

You may be wondering if you are a good candidate for plastic surgery. This depends on a number of factors, including age, medical history, and personal body image. I will discuss in detail the various procedures available and the difficulties that may arise for each age group.

COSMETIC SURGERY MAY SEEM LIKE A GAMBLE, BUT IT DOESN'T HAVE TO BE

I will also discuss the options for men in the area of body sculpting. The number of surgical procedures available for men has grown tremendously over the past few years, and as cosmetic surgery becomes more common, I anticipate this growth continuing. There are special considerations and procedures that men should be aware of, and I will detail those in a subsequent chapter.

There are several procedures that I will specifically address in this book. One of them is breast augmentation. This is one of the top five procedures performed each year across the country, and it is also one of the procedures that can go very badly when done by an untrained physician.

But what if you already had a cosmetic procedure and were very disappointed with the results? I spend a full chapter (chapter 6) discussing when and how you can consider a revision or correction and what you can realistically expect from that experience.

Cosmetic surgery may seem like a gamble, but it doesn't have to be. A knowledgeable patient with realistic expectations and confidence in their surgeon can have a predictable, fabulous outcome. Come along with me and I'll show you how.

NOTES

_____

_____

_____

_____

_____

_____

_____

_____

_____

_____

_____

_____

_____

_____

_____

_____

_____

_____

_____

_____

_____

_____

_____

_____

_____

_____

_____

_____

_____

NOTES

_____

_____

_____

_____

_____

_____

_____

_____

_____

_____

_____

_____

_____

_____

_____

_____

_____

_____

_____

_____

_____

_____

_____

_____

_____

_____

_____

_____

_____

NOTES

_____

_____

_____

_____

_____

_____

_____

_____

_____

_____

_____

_____

_____

_____

_____

_____

_____

_____

_____

_____

_____

_____

_____

_____

_____

_____

_____

_____

"BEAUTY LASTS FIVE
MINUTES. MAYBE LONGER
IF YOU HAVE A GOOD
PLASTIC SURGEON."
— TIA CARRERE

CHAPTER 2
Finding a Doctor

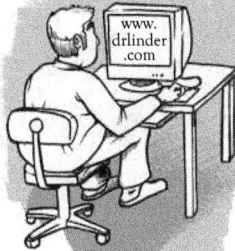

"People see you as an object, not as a person, and they project a set of expectations onto you. People who don't have it think beauty is a blessing, but actually it sets you apart."

— *Candace Bergen*

One of the first questions that comes to mind when an individual contemplates having cosmetic surgery is, "What do I want to have done and why?" While this may seem like an easy question to answer, it really isn't, and the answer varies significantly from patient to patient. Not only must you know what areas of your body you want to address, but you must also know why.

Examining your own motivations can either help you have confidence in your decision and in your doctor, or it can serve as a dire warning. For example, are you feeling pressured by a friend, partner or relative to have a procedure done? Do you think that plastic surgery will mend your marriage, help you get a better job, or give you perfection? If these "solutions" are anywhere in your thought process,

I would strongly encourage you to step back and think long and hard before proceeding.

While plastic surgery can do many things for your outward appearance, it cannot fix the problems in your life. Every day people come to me and request procedure after procedure, chasing some illusion of perfection that simply doesn't exist. They become plastic surgery "junkies" with unrealistic hopes and expectations. Moving around the tissue on your body will not have a lasting effect on your psychological state of being, nor will it be the door of opportunity to a new and different life. This is because it changes only the outside; it doesn't change who you are.

Having said that, I'll add that if you feel self-conscious about the small but noticeable signs of aging, have lost significant weight, or would like to look less tired and more like the "you" that you remember, there are a plethora of cosmetic procedures that can help you regain your self-confidence. The difference between these reasons for plastic surgery and those that I listed earlier is that you just want to be a better version of yourself, not a different person, and that is what I want for each of my patients.

> MOST PEOPLE WANT TO PROJECT AN IMAGE THAT REFLECTS THE WAY THEY SEE THEMSELVES

Most people want to project an image that reflects the way they see themselves: as a vibrant, energetic individual. But many times that person will look in the mirror and see a much older person staring back. Often they come into my office and ask, "Where did all the wrinkles come from, and why are my cheeks sliding down my face? And what's up with the turkey neck? I don't understand why I feel better than I have in years, yet my breasts look like I'm 80!"

When reacting to the aging process, emotions range from mild disappointment to panic and sometimes even outright anger as a feeling of helplessness sets in. You don't have to resign yourself to feeling old every time you look in the mirror. These days, people in their 40s and 50s are more vibrant than ever, and they want their outside appearance to match the inside.

I feel I should warn you that once you have made the decision to have plastic surgery people you will expect to support your decision may have a very difficult time accepting it. Friends and family can be a great source of comfort, but they can also be a tremendous source of stress during the decision-making process. You may find that your children, parents, or even spouse are not in agreement with your decision to surgically alter your looks. They may accuse you of being vain or hint that you've gone off the deep end.

I encourage you to look behind their reactions and understand the real emotions at work. For your family, the idea of you going into surgery for several hours is a scary thing. They are thinking, "What if something happens?" "What if you are horribly disfigured or even die?" "And how can you afford to 'waste' the money for this?" Please talk to your family and let them express these emotions and concerns. This is your chance to educate them and help them understand what you are doing. In the end, this is your decision, your body, and your well-being at stake. While your family may not agree with your decision at first, hopefully, they will come to understand that this is what you want, and they will support you.

There will also be individuals, such as friends and coworkers, who may surprise you with their reactions. They may feel threatened that you will soon look younger and more vibrant than they do. Snide comments and rude talk around the office are not uncommon obstacles for patients to face both before and after surgery. Here again, look at the emotions that lie behind their actions. Jealousy and envy are powerful demons that will try to undermine your new sense of self-worth. While there isn't much you can do about other people, you can be ready for their reactions and prepare yourself to withstand the gossip.

Once you have definitely decided to move ahead with a procedure, and you are aware and comfortable with your own motivations, the most important decision you will now make is choosing which doctor will perform your surgery.

Choosing a Doctor

I cannot lead you to think that finding the right doctor is an easy process. The medical world can be intimidating and hard to understand for anyone approaching this for the first time. However, this is your body and your life and you deserve the utmost respect from any physician you allow to approach your body. You should know every possible detail about that doctor's training and experience. To help you on your journey, I have provided a worksheet, found at the end of this chapter that you can take along with you on your consultations. This will help ensure that you cover all the basics and are able to compare physicians.

I know the concept of comparing physicians may seem a bit foreign to you, but it is very important. You want to be sure you will get the best results possible and be cared for properly during recovery. It is to your long-term benefit to keep looking until you find a doctor who has the right combination of training and experience in the procedure you are contemplating.

To get started, we will go over some of the basic qualifications that every single doctor you visit should have. This will help you narrow down the choices to a few physicians with whom you will want to set up initial consultations. I recommend that you visit and talk to at least three doctors before making any decision, and if none of them seems right, keep looking. You never regret the mistake you don't make. So take your time and be sure.

Basic Qualifications

You will probably begin your search, as most people do, on the phone or over the Internet. There are a few very basic criteria that your doctor must possess before you make an appointment, and these can't be compromised or negated in any way.

Qualification #1: Board Certification of Your Doctor

Board certification may sound like a simple thing. After all, you've seen the fancy diplomas framed on your general physician's walls, right? Well that doesn't mean much in the area of cosmetic surgery. Many people are shocked to find that virtually any doctor with an MD behind their name can do cosmetic procedures. There are no rules requiring special training or additional experience on the doctor's part. This means that any emergency room physician, gynecologist, or internist can perform cosmetic procedures.

LOOK FOR A DOCTOR WHO IS A DIPLOMAT OR BOARD CERTIFIED BY THE AMERICAN BOARD OF PLASTIC SURGERY

So, how do you know that the doctor with whom you are speaking is qualified to do the procedure you want? Look for a doctor who is recognized by the American Board of Medical Specialties (ABMS) and is a diplomat or board certified by the American Board of Plastic Surgery (ABPS). The ABPS has very strict guidelines for granting certification.

Verifying certification can get very confusing if your doctor insists he or she is board certified in cosmetic surgery but doesn't specifically say that he or she is ABMS certified in plastic surgery. I will warn you now that if this happens you should look elsewhere. There are many sound-alike medical boards out there, and coming from a doctor, those credentials might give the impression that your doctor is as highly qualified as one certified by the American Board of Plastic Surgery. The truth is that any group of doctors can get together and create their own certification board. Many of these boards apply to the ABMS for membership, but to date, only a select few have ever been accepted. More than 100 boards have been rejected but are still out there, operating under their own guidelines and requirements.

When doctors skirt the certification question or give the impression that they are just as qualified as board-certified plastic surgeons, in my opinion, they are being unethical. They are intentionally misleading patients about their level of training. Be very sure that the doctor you choose doesn't fall into this category but is a bona-fide board-certified plastic surgeon. You can rest assured that doctors who have taken the extra time to go through this rigorous certification process did not take shortcuts in their education and training. And, they will also not take shortcuts during your surgery, either.

You may think that this is overkill, especially if you want just a nip here or a tuck there. While experience and training are very important for a good result, they are even more important if something goes wrong. The additional training and experience gives a board-certified plastic surgeon a distinct advantage over other doctors. They have an additional seven to thirteen years of experience performing these procedures day in and day out. They weren't taking out a gallbladder yesterday and then doing a breast lift today. When there are unexpected complications, or something unusual is encountered during surgery, it is the more experienced surgeon whom you want in charge. He or she may not only ensure that the procedure still has the possibility of a good outcome, he or she may also save your life.

ASK WHICH CERTIFICATIONS YOUR DOCTOR HAS RECEIVED

Another question you will want to ask your doctor is where they received their training. Any good doctor will readily give you a list of where they received their medical degree, where they did their residencies, and in what facilities they have practiced since that time.

The normal career path for any doctor is to graduate medical school and then complete a residency, which is practical, on-the-job training in a hospital setting. The physicians who wish to become board certified in a particular field, such as plastic surgery, then do a second residency focusing solely on that area of practice. It is in this second residency that the doctor receives intensive training by experienced plastic surgeons. The doctor can then choose to attain special certifications in specific procedures. Ask which certifications your doctor has received and what techniques they use. It is important for any doctor to remain aware of the newest advancements in his or her area of expertise and to be knowledgeable of new technology and techniques. Plastic surgeons are required to maintain 150 hours of continued medical education(CME) every three years. This is important because these educational hours help to keep the surgeon current with new practices.

You will also want to ask if the doctor performs the surgery you are requesting on a daily or weekly basis and what percentage of the overall business is devoted to doing this procedure. While they may tell you that they do a particular type of surgery an average of once a week, it may only be a very small percentage of the overall practice. You have to remember that they call a doctor's business a "practice" for a reason. You have to do a procedure over and over to be good at it. And you want the best that you can get.

In order to get specific answers, you must ask specific questions. Don't be afraid that the doctor will mind; we don't—at least the reputable ones don't. In fact, I love it when a patient asks about my training. It gives me the opportunity to let them know they are getting a well-qualified doctor who they can give their full trust. It also shows me that I am dealing with a person who is willing to educate him or herself and take an active role in his or her own recovery. I find that this type of patient usually has the best outcome because we are working as a team.

Qualification #2: Certification of the Surgery Center

Where will your surgery be performed? You may assume that it will be in the hospital, but that is not necessarily so. In fact, most plastic surgery and cosmetic procedures are performed on an outpatient basis in an ambulatory surgical center. Smaller procedures may even be performed in the doctor's office.

Years ago, when the baby boomers were toddlers, hospitals were inspected, reviewed, and given a seal of approval. Ambulatory surgical centers didn't even exist, so now that many procedures are performed in these new facilities, most of them will voluntarily choose to undergo an accreditation process to assure their patients' safety. The American Board of Plastic Surgery requires that all diplomats operate only in certified or state-licensed ambulatory centers. This is an additional safety net for the patient.

Accrediting organizations verify that national standards are met and maintained within the surgical environment. They review policies and procedures, safety, equipment, the handling of blood, and medications. The organization verifies that the surgeon has hospital privileges should an emergency necessitating the patient be transferred to a hospital occur. It ensures that the facility keeps adequate records, has an emergency plan and emergency procedures in place, and verifies the credentials of all staff members. The accrediting organization also certifies the types of anesthesia that may be administered in the facility and under what circumstances.

For example, the American Association for Accreditaion of Ambulatory Surgery Facilities, Inc. (AAAASF-also known as Quad-A) classifies ambulatory facilities into three levels: A, B, or C. In Class A–approved facilities, procedures may only be performed under local or topical anesthesia without IV sedation. Class A/B facilities may administer local anesthesia as well as IV sedation. Class A/B/C facilities may administer local, IV sedation, or general anesthesia.

Be sure your facility, at the minimum, is state licensed and Quad A certified. If Medicare will be involved in reimbursement (as is the case in some reconstructive surgeries and procedures), then the facility must also be Medicare approved.

Qualification #3: Capable and Certified Staff at the Facility

Next to your surgeon, the most important member of the medical team will be the anesthesiologist. In my practice, I use only board-certified anesthesiologists. These individuals are also MDs. While there may be others on the medical team who are capable of administering anesthesia, the additional education, training, and experience of a board-certified anesthesiologist give the patient enormous protection. Of all the things that can go wrong in any surgery, anesthesia problems can be the most life threatening. The combination and type of anesthesia can be different for each patient, based on the specific type of procedure or procedures being done, age, and overall health.

The surgeon and anesthesiologist work in tandem to assure that there are no reactions to the anesthesia and that the patient is neither under- or overmedicated. This can be very tricky business, and many times adjustments must be made on the spot, especially if it appears there may be a problem or if the surgery lasts longer than predicted. These adjustments need the expertise and skill that only experience brings. A well-qualified anesthesiologist should be able to prevent "recall" of the surgery and to reduce incidence of postoperative nausea and/or vomiting with new medications such as Zofran.

> BE SURE THE FACILITY YOU CHOOSE IS A SPARKLING EXAMPLE OF CLEANLINESS.

The rest of the medical team should consist of a director of nursing, circulating nurses, and scrub technicians. Ask if you can talk with or meet these people. You want to know their experience with the facility and with the doctor who will be performing your surgery. You will also pick up a lot of clues about the operation of the facility from the attitude and demeanor of the staff. Are they respectful and open, or is there an underlying tension? Ask if you can tour the surgical facility and be sure to take notes. Is it clean and tidy? Are the surgical areas and instruments kept sterile? Disorganization within the facility could indicate the same level of disorganization inside the surgical area as well. The possibility of infection, and complications from an infection, are too big of risk. Be sure the facility you choose is a sparkling example of cleanliness.

Qualification #4: References

Ask the doctor for several references from patients who've had the same procedure you are thinking about having. Call each one, and ask them about their experience. These people can tell you of their experience with the doctor and staff, the recovery process and how they feel about their end result.

While this may take some time, it is worth the effort to get all of your questions answered and alleviate any reservations you may still have. Once you have called all the doctors on your list and completed the qualification worksheet, you are ready to move on to the initial consult. Here again, I have included a worksheet at the end of this chapter to take with you to aid in gathering as much information as possible to assist you in making your final decision.

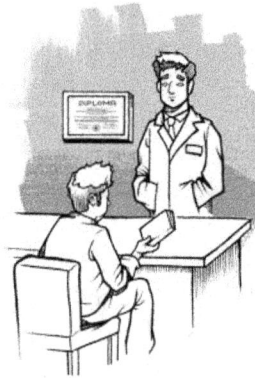

INITIAL CONSULT

By now, you should have narrowed your list of physicians down to the top three candidates, who can be ranked as A, B, and C. These are the doctors with whom you should set up your initial consultations. The following are items you should consider and take notes on in order to review and compare later:

#1: Physical Environment

Is the office neat and tidy? Does it feel warm and welcoming? Does the staff greet you calmly, or do they seem stressed and short tempered? As you sit and wait, notice how the front-office staff answers the phone, interacts with other patients, and goes about working. If there are other patients waiting, take the opportunity to ask of their experiences.

How long is the right amount of time to wait? Ideally, you would think none. If you make an appointment, you should see the doctor at that specified time and not wait at all. But plastic surgery is different than most other specialties. Rarely do patients have so many questions or concerns as they do when they are altering their appearance. You want a doctor who will take the time to answer all of your questions rather than rushing to his next appointment. You will know generally by the office environment if the doctor is merely overbooking to get as many patients through as possible or if he/she is spending quality time with each patient. If they are taking quality time, then waiting a little bit longer is not necessarily a bad thing.

#2: Office Staff

When you are taken back for your appointment, does the staff treat you with courtesy and respect? Are you going to spend time with the doctor, or do you find that you spend most of your time talking to a nurse? On the first consultation, you should expect to spend most of your time with the doctor. The doctor should be the one to answer your questions and concerns, not a staff member. Do not allow the staff or the doctor to cut your visit short. Be sure that all of your questions are answered.

> DON'T BE AFRAID THAT YOU ARE ASKING TOO MANY QUESTIONS.

#3: The Doctor

Once you get to sit down face to face with the doctor, evaluate your conversation as honestly as possible. Does the doctor listen to what you want and what your goals are? Some doctors may hear your first comments about what you want to change, then immediately start offering solutions. But you want to be sure they hear and understand what you want for your body, not what they think you need. As you talk, evaluate whether the doctor understands what is motivating you to make these changes. The doctor may be able to offer different and better solutions once the entire picture is understood.

Don't be afraid that you are asking too many questions. That is what the initial consultation is about. Continue to ask until every question you have is thoroughly answered. Don't let the doctor get away with technical jargon, either. Ask him to explain your procedure in layman's terms, and expect to receive quality printed brochures and patient information fliers to take with you.

In order to have a good consultation and an eventual good outcome, you must be upfront and honest with your doctor about every aspect of your health. This includes any current or former medical problems, drugs or even supplements you might be taking, and activities in which you are involved. The doctor must know about your lifestyle and what kind of individual you are in order to give accurate predictions of your surgery and recovery. It is a surprise to most patients that something as minor as taking a particular over-the-counter supplement can lessen their chances of a good outcome, but it is true, so be sure to include every aspect of your health in the initial evaluation.

Most doctors will have before-and-after photos. It is easy to get excited when you look at these because they are usually the best-case scenarios. The individuals in the photos look great and had a good outcome, or they wouldn't be in the book in the first place. But, there are several questions you must ask about them. Are the photos actual patients of the doctor doing the consult? If not, ask to see photos of his actual patients. He should have plenty of these. Do these patients look the way you want to look after your procedure? If not, or if you don't like some of the results, discuss these with the doctor. You want them to have a clear understanding of your expectations, not only what you want, but what you don't want as well.

#4: Get a Written Fee Quote

Once you discuss your procedure in depth, talk about the cost and get a quote in writing. This helps tremendously when comparing each doctor, and, again, ask questions. One important thing to remember about fees is that, while you will pay a somewhat higher fee for a board-certified doctor, the most expensive is not always the best. Some doctors charge exorbitant fees because they know that some people equate price with quality. Be warned: some of these high-priced doctors are not board certified. So don't let a higher price alone convince you that you're getting something spectacular. Cost is only one factor in your decision-making process. And once again, if the fee is way below the rest of your quotes from doctors in the same geographic area, then you have to ask yourself, "Why?"

#5: Overall Impression

As soon as you leave the doctor's office, take a few minutes to write notes on your overall impression of the consult. Are the doctor and his staff who you want guiding you through this process? Did you feel pushed to have more procedures than you planned on when you walked in initially? Did they rush you to make a decision and get you into their schedule? Rank your consultations on a scale from one to five and compare them. Even if you think you have found your doctor on the first visit, I would encourage you to go ahead and keep your appointments with the other doctors. They may offer additional solutions or raise issues that this doctor didn't, and you might like them and their staff better.

#6: Doctor's Record

One last area you will want to check is the doctor's malpractice record. This should be one of the questions you ask him in person, and then verify his answer with your state board of insurance.

While this type of doctor hunting takes precious time away from your family and from work, it is still very important to follow through and make sure you are getting the best doctor possible. The more knowledge you aquire, the more likely it is that you will have a great result.

> THE MORE KNOWLEDGE YOU AQUIRE, THE MORE LIKELY IT IS THAT YOU WILL HAVE A GREAT RESULT.

SCREENING WORKSHEET

After you've done your research, you will want to prepare yourself as best as you can for your appointments. It is absolutely vital that you take a worksheet of all the important questions with you, so that you and the doctor can go through it point by point and not leave anything out. This will be the most valuable tool that you will have to assist you in making an informed, educated decision.

• Name of doctor.

  _____

• Specialty?

  _____

• Is the doctor a diplomat of the American Board of Plastic Surgery?

  yes _____   no _____

  If not, why? _____

• Number of procedures performed per year of the specific procedure that you are looking to have done. For example, if you're having breast augmentation, how many augmentations has the doctor performed
  per week?   _____
  per month? _____
  per year?   _____

• Number of years in practice? _____

• Malpractice lawsuits? Number of lawsuits _____,
  and outcomes. _____

- Surgical approach used for the procedure that you are considering. (This is very important; there are various techniques that can be used for each procedure. For example, for breast augmentation there are different kinds of incisions: peri-areolar, through the belly button, under the armpit, over the muscle, under the muscle, etc. You need to know which technique is the safest and which will provide you with the best possible results.)

  _____

  _____

  _____

- Photographs. Review as many before-and-after photos as possible. Be sure to look at the height, weight, and body dimensions of each patient and what the results look like after. Do they look "done," or are they natural looking? Does the doctor have the ability to make you look the way you want to look?

  _____

  _____

  _____

- Anesthesia. Does the surgeon use the services of a nurse anesthetist or an anesthesiologist that is a diplomat of the American Board of Anesthesiology? This is very important; there is a difference.

  _____

  _____

  What is the anesthesiologist's name? _____

  Number of years in practice? _____

  Malpractice record? _____

- Where will the surgery be performed? Is it in the office, at an ambulatory surgical center, or at the hospital?

  _____

  Is the facility licensed?   _____
  Is it Medicare approved?   _____
  Is it state certified?   _____

- Will the procedure be done on an outpatient or inpatient basis?

  _____

  If done at an outpatient facility, what is the reciprocity agreement with nearby hospitals for emergency purposes?

  _____

  Name of Hospital: _____

  Is there a contract with paramedics and ambulance services for emergencies?

  _____

- Revisions. What will your responsibility be for revisions?

  _____

  Will you be responsible for operating room fees? _____
  Anesthesia fees? _____
  Or for a total fee once again? _____

- What is your financial responsibility if something goes wrong after your initial surgery? _____

  If you develop an infection, have a deflation of an implant, or develop hypertrophic scarring? _____

- Nursing staff and surgical scrub technicians. All of these people will be a part of your surgery. Are they certified and/or licensed?

  _____

  ICU certified? _____
  How many years have they been with the doctor and at the facility?

  _____

- Postoperative care. What will the follow-up appointments be like?

  _____

  How many follow-up visits will you need to make during your recovery process? _____

  When will your stitches (sutures) be removed? _____
  By whom? _____

- Physician coverage and after-hours contact. How will you reach the surgeon after-hours if you have an issue?

  _____

  _____

  If your doctor is not available, how is coverage for him/her handled? _____

- What should you expect during the recovery process?

  _____

  _____

  _____

  Will you receive a list of do's and don'ts to have on hand while you're recovering?

  _____

NOTES

_____

_____

_____

_____

_____

_____

_____

_____

_____

_____

_____

_____

_____

_____

_____

_____

_____

_____

_____

_____

_____

_____

_____

_____

_____

_____

_____

_____

_____

_____

_____

_____

NOTES

_____
_____
_____
_____
_____
_____
_____
_____
_____
_____
_____
_____
_____
_____
_____
_____
_____
_____
_____
_____
_____
_____
_____
_____
_____
_____
_____

"THE WORD "**PLASTIC**"
DERIVES FROM THE
GREEK PLASTIKOS
MEANING TO MOLD
OR TO SHAPE."

CHAPTER 3
The Stages of Life for Women

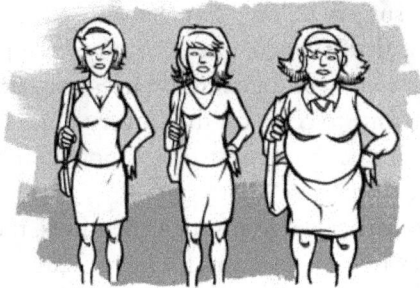

"You start out happy that you have no hips or boobs. All of a sudden you get them, and it feels sloppy. Then just when you start liking them, they start drooping."

– Cindy Crawford

There are as many different reasons for contemplating cosmetic surgery as there are individuals in the world. Body sculpting is becoming more and more popular as people realize that they do not have to sit back and merely accept the effects of aging and circumstances. They can do something about it.

But how do you know if you are a good candidate for a specific procedure? Just because a friend or a family member had a procedure and enjoyed a great result, doesn't mean that you can or should do the same. Each procedure must fit your body type, age range, and specific health issues. Since no two people are alike, you should never assume that you can have the same outcome as the next person. Plastic surgery is specific for each individual, unlike most other surgeries. The results show. They have to be tailored to each specific patient.

Some people think getting breast implants or a nose job is much like the old Mr. Potato Head toys. You have one set of lips, nose, or eyes, and they all fit no matter who you put them on. Nothing could be further from the truth! Because we each have different body types, goals, and medical issues, there is no way to make these surgeries identical, nor should there be.

You deserve a surgery tailored to meet your goals and circumstances, one that will take into account all the possibilities and options given your special set of circumstances. Any doctor who is not willing to take the time to conform the surgery to your body, rather than conforming to what he wants to do, is not worth your time or hard-earned money.

As women, in particular, go through their lives, there are specific life events that may trigger the desire for plastic surgery. These include childbearing, massive weight loss, and premature aging. We will go over these different life stages individually and discuss specific procedures that you may be contemplating if you fall into one of these categories.

Men age differently and are held to different societal standards, but there is one thing that all of my patients have in common: they want to look and feel better about themselves. More and more men are turning to plastic surgery to get their self-confidence back and reduce the signs of aging.

Men and women have gender-specific needs and concerns regarding plastic surgery. For that reason, I will deal with them separately. In this chapter, we will discuss the procedures and concerns that affect most women. In the next chapter, we will discuss body sculpting for men.

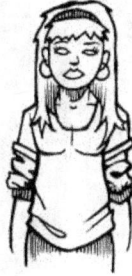

LIFE SEGMENT ONE: TEENAGERS

In general, young women under the age of eighteen should not undergo plastic surgery. I feel strongly that as surgeons we have an ethical responsibility to make sure that teenagers are both physically and psychologically ready for an operation, especially breast enhancement surgery.

Often it is difficult for a very young woman to perceive and comprehend all the ramifications and consequences of making a life-altering change so early on. What sounded like a great idea at sixteen may be completely regrettable at twenty-six. For this reason, I am very careful. The Hippocratic Oath that all doctors abide by says, "First, do no harm." This is especially true with plastic surgery. While the patient may physically heal and look great, if the decision for surgery is made before the patient is really ready, the psychological damage can last a lifetime.

There are rare exceptions to this rule, and I see a few of them each year. These exceptions include young women with severe congenital breast deformity, which is the absence of one breast. For example, the right breast may be a full C cup and sagging, while the left breast is an A cup and not sagging. While this sounds horrific, and it is to those patients who suffer from it, it is correctable.

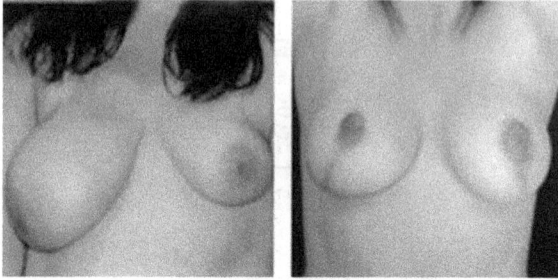

Patient had a 34E breast on the right with severe sagginess and a full 34B breast on the left. Her surgery consisted of a breast reduction on the right and a 320 cc saline implant on the left with a breast lift.

These young patients are usually brought into my office by parents who are concerned that the deformity is causing extreme distress to their daughters. During the high school years, a woman's sense of self and her self confidence are still forming. This kind of physical deformity can lead to insecurity, depression, and fear of socializing, all of which can irreparably damage a young woman's self-esteem.

Even though it is obvious that this is a situation that would need correction, surgeons are still very careful. We must be confident that the young woman is mature enough to understand the procedure and consent to it. We must also have the consent of the parents, as well as specific documentation and agreement from endocrinologists and pediatricians. Only at this point will we do the procedure, which will give the patient similar size and symmetry of her breasts and will allow her to feel more comfortable with her body.

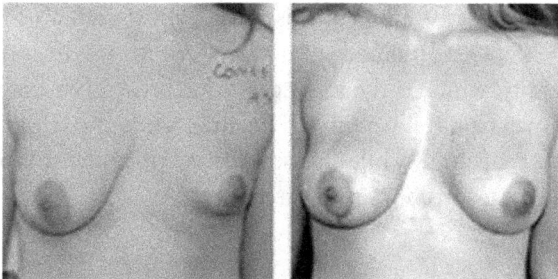

Patient had a 34C breast with severe sagginess on the right with a 34A breast on the left. Surgery consisted of a breast lift on the right and a 390 cc saline implant placed under the muscle on the left.

In these young women, we also sometimes see what is known as Tubular Breast Deformities. Approximately one to two percent of young women that come in for consultation have this condition. This deformity can be a very distressing problem because the breasts appear abnormal in both size and shape.

Characteristics of a tubular breast deformity usually include fat that herniates, or intrudes, into the nipple areolar complex making it look puffy and distended. Flattening of the lower pole of the breast with a loss or absence of breast tissue causes a flattening of the entire lower portion of the breast so that it doesn't appear round in shape and is, in effect, tubular. The fold at the bottom of the breast (inframammary fold) is often either poorly defined or not defined at all. These women usually require breast augmentation surgery with release of the lower portion of the breast tissue in order to recreate a normal shape and roundness to the bottom of their breasts.

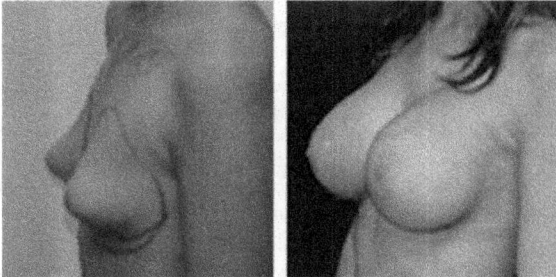

Patient had a conical shape to her breasts with herniation of fat into the nipple areolar complexes and a flattening of the bottom of her breasts. She underwent breast augmentation with 425 cc high profile saline implants in the dual plane and complete release of the lower portion of her breasts. She was required to wear an upper pole compression band for four weeks to help drop the implants and round out the bottom of her breasts.

Tubular breasts can appear in either one or both breasts. They can also be associated with Poland syndrome, in which the patient has an absence of the complete, or portions of, the pectoralis major muscle and a very small breast, causing severe chest deformity. These patients usually will require augmentation alone, however, if they also have loose, saggy skin they may require a breast lift at the same time to achieve the desired result.

Correcting a tubular breast deformity can be very difficult. In the past, implants were usually placed above the muscle in order to recreate a more round appearance of the breast, but at this stage in my practice I prefer to place the implants, most of the time at least, half under the muscle and half over and completely release the lower portion of the breast to create a beautiful, rounder, more natural appearing shape while reducing the visibility of the implant bag edge along the inner aspect of the chest area. It is important to be aware that Tubular Breast Deformity patients can also have significant amounts of stretching that occurs with implants, which can lead to increased stretch marks along the breasts.

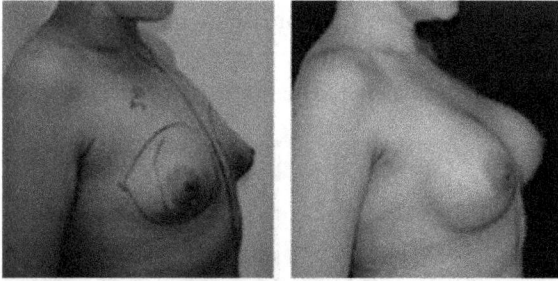

Patient had loss of fullness to the lower portion of her breasts with conical shape and herniation of tissue into the nipple areolar complexes. She had an augmentation mammoplasty procedure with 420 cc implants and release of the fold.

Some young women may also experience a condition where they endure massive breasts. We see patients occasionally who are under the age of eighteen with enormous breast hypertrophy or gigantic breasts (gigantomastia). Again, these patients arrive with a parent, and while they suffer the same extreme psychological distress as the aforementioned patients, they also suffer from significant physical discomfort. Many have severe back pain and neck problems due to the massive weight of their breasts. Many times the breasts are so large that bra straps will cause permanent grooving in the young woman's shoulders. These women can also suffer from rashes and sores, as the large areas of skin press against one another.

We as doctors still like to wait, if possible, until the young woman is at least eighteen in order to decrease the likelihood that the breasts will grow back and the surgery will have to be performed again. However, if the symptoms are severe, we will perform a breast reduction, which involves removal of breast tissue and skin to alleviate the symptoms and reduce their massive weight. No patient should suffer from these types of horrible symptoms, regardless of age.

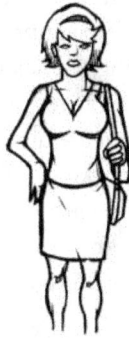

LIFE SEGMENT TWO: YOUNG WOMEN AGES 18-30

Women between the ages of eighteen and thirty who have not breast-fed or experienced pregnancy may be very good candidates for breast enhancement surgery. Many times these women are unhappy with the appearance of their breasts (breast dysphoria), or their breasts are simply small (breast hypoplasia).

Normally, the breast implants are placed using a technique called dual plane. This means that the inner portion of the implant is placed under the muscle and the outer portion of the implant is placed above the muscle. We use this technique because it gives an excellent, natural-looking result.

If you have ever seen a woman whose cleavage is defined by two very obvious edges of round implants, it is a unattactive result. The best result is evident when no one but that woman knows that anything was ever done. That is our goal and our reasoning for using the dual plane technique.

One word of caution for women who fall within this age group: the fact that your skin has not been softened or stretched by pregnancy, or by age in general, can limit the size of implant that is used. Your skin is thick, and stretching it too far can produce unsightly stretch marks. Also, the muscles of your chest are firm and tight. This can mean that you will wind up with rounder, harder breasts, at least early on.

Be aware of these limitations and issues, and set realistic goals. The idea behind breast augmentation is to achieve a symmetrical, proportional, and very natural appearance. This adds to a woman's sexuality and feeling of well-being, especially when her goals are realistic and the anticipated surgery result is achieved.

The women in this age group are also good candidates for small liposuction procedures. Small pockets of fat that are resistant to diet and exercise can be removed with a good result. Rarely do these women need any sort of significant procedures, unless they have a congenital deformity of some sort or have experienced a large amount of weight loss.

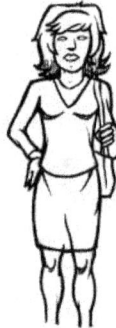

LIFE STAGE THREE WOMEN AGES 30-50

(NO HISTORY OF PREGNANCY, WEIGHT LOSS, OR BREAST-FEEDING)

Women in this life stage usually do very well during cosmetic procedures and are especially good candidates for breast augmentation. Their skin and tissues have softened at least somewhat over time potentially due to weight fluctuation. Once again, making the implants accent the woman's body and look as natural as possible is the goal. Every woman wants to look beautiful and sexy without feeling matronly or overdone.

One thing that many people do not realize is that not only do breasts sag downward over time, the also spread out. This produces a wide or "matronly looking" breast, especially when viewed from the side. A younger woman's breast usually has a round and shapely appearance from the side. But many women, as they reach middle age, lose this youthful appearance and cease wearing any clothing that exposes the outside edges of their breasts.

This is why my practice uses what is called a high-profile saline implant for these types of patients. "High-profile" means that the implants have more fullness and projection. They project

> MY GOAL IS TO HELP A WOMAN LOOK SEXY AND FEEL GREAT

further from the chest and look a little rounder, giving a less matronly appearance from the side. They are not as wide and give the woman a beautiful, tapered appearance. They are similar to a gorgeous Vera Wang wedding dress that is professionally cut and shaped on the side so as to accentuate the woman's breasts, not cover them up. My goal is to help a woman look sexy and feel great, and in my opinion, these are some of the most beautiful implants in the world.

As with the previous age group, women in this classification are also good candidates for liposuction and limited facial procedures. There is usually little else necessary to restore a feeling of youth and beauty.

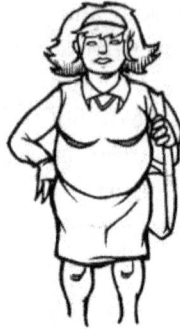

LIFE SEGMENT FOUR: WOMEN AGES 30-50

(SIGNIFICANT HISTORY OF WEIGHT LOSS, MULTIPLE PREGNANCIES, BREAST-FEEDING)

Women in this age group who have experienced circumstances such as massive weight loss, multiple pregnancies, and breast-feeding often find that over time, not only do they experience a loss of volume, but they also experience a great deal of sagging of the breasts. Many times, in conjunction with breast implants to replace that volume, they also must have a breast lift (mastopexy). These operations can be done at the same time if you have an experienced, board-certified plastic surgeon. Occasionally, doctors need to stage the operations (having the operation in 2 surgeries rather than one), but this is usually due to specific health issues that require us to do them separately. Most of the time, the breast lift and augmentation will be performed together.

If you are uncertain as to whether you need a breast lift or not, there is an easy way to tell. Stand up and find the crease under your breast with your fingers. If your nipple rests below this crease then you will probably need a breast lift.

Performing a breast lift is often an absolute necessity. Unfortunately, many patients come into my office asking for this procedure after having had a breast augmentation elsewhere. They are unhappy because the surgeon gave them exactly what they asked for. That's right: exactly what they asked for. They wanted a breast augmentation and got it. But what they needed was a breast lift **and** augmentation.

In the immortal words of Mick Jagger, "You can't always get what you want, but if you try sometime, you just might find you get what you need." And so it is in my practice. On numerous occasions I have had a patient request an augmentation, yet refuse a needed breast lift because they didn't want scars. I explain to them that if you have excess skin, and just have an augmentation without the lift; it will lead to a "rock in a sock" appearance. The implant will end up at the bottom of the breast a short time after surgery and will make the skin sag even worse.

I always advise this type of patient that if she isn't willing to have the lift, then the augmentation will be a disaapointment. If the patient still insists, I refuse to do the surgery. If you have excess skin and go to a surgeon who tells you that you can get away with just an augmentation, seek a second opinion from a board-certified plastic surgeon or you most likely end up unhappy with your result.

THE IMPORTANT THING TO REMEMBER IS TO HAVE REALISTIC EXPECTATIONS.

The important thing to remember is to have realistic expectations. If you absolutely do not want the scars associated with a breast lift, that's fine and understandable, but I would advise you that it is much better not to have any procedure at all rather than have one with which you will be unhappy.

Women in this group often have some of the more extensive procedures, such as tummy tucks, belt lipectomy, and full face-lifts. Childbearing and massive weight loss are both hard on the body, and the consequences can look less than appealing. While many of these procedures produce the biggest scars, I find that patients in this category are usually the happiest with the results.

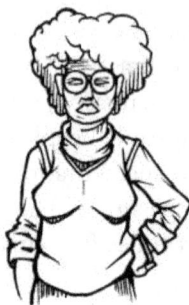

LIFE SEGMENT FIVE: WOMEN OVER 50
(LOSS OF BREAST TISSUE AND SAGGING OF THE BREASTS AND BODY)

These women usually require both a breast lift and augmentation at the same time. If you are in this category, it is extremely important that you do not go with implants that are too large. As we age, the skin thins out and loses its elasticity. The older we are, the greater the tendency for our skin to sag. If a woman opts for large implants, gravity will pull these with horrendous results, especially if she doesn't always wear a supportive bra. You could easily end up looking worse than you did before you had the procedure.

Many women at this stage of their lives are coming back to replace implants that were put in many years ago. This is called breast revision surgery and is one of my specialties. I personally love doing this procedure because it is a challenge. Revising breast implants from the past can be very difficult, but rewarding as well.

Sometimes the women that I see in my office have had silicone implants that have been in place for twenty, thirty, or even forty years. Most of the time, these implants have ruptured or dissolved and are nothing but goop. All of this material must be removed from the patient.

Years ago, Dow Corning implants actually had five patches that adhered the implant to the chest wall and kept it in place. These patches must be carefully stripped off the chest wall. A board—certified plastic surgeon can accomplish this safely, without venturing near your pleural space or your lung. All of the sticky, gooey silicone must be removed and the shell of the implant bag taken out. The scar tissue (the capsule) that forms around an implant has usually calcified into a hard chalk-like substance. This must also be removed and sent, along with the old silicone implants, to pathology for diagnostic purposes. Patients who have previously had silicone implants usually replace them with the same.

Women in this category are most often bothered by the appearance of their face as it wrinkles and their skin as it sags. Loss of volume in the cheek area can give a sunken and hollow look that ages the face as well. There are many procedures that can help these areas and restore a more youthful appearance. It is best to consult with your doctor and find the right procedure or mix of procedures that work for you.

MEDICAL ISSUES

One other area that you must think about when determining if you are a good candidate for plastic surgery is your overall health. Many medical conditions and life choices may affect your recovery and overall result. Being aware of these, and informing your doctor at the first consultation, will make your procedure much easier and your recovery faster.

Smoking

Many smokers assume that all doctors are against smoking as a rule, which is true on one level. No doctor wants you to engage in an activity that is known to harm you. With plastic surgery, smoking is even more hazardous than normal. Nicotine restricts the flow of blood in your blood vessels. This includes the tiny capillaries in the skin. It is these small capillaries that we depend on after plastic surgery to help heal wounds quickly, with as little scarring as possible.

Smokers tend to have poorer blood flow to their skin in general and shouldn't expect as good a result as nonsmokers have. That's just a fact. Some plastic surgeons will even refuse to do face-lifts on longtime smokers because they know the chances of a good result are

AS A PATIENT, YOU MUST BE OPEN AND HONEST WITH YOUR SURGEON.

much lower, and they do not wish to harm the patient. When there is lack of blood flow, the skin around the incision can sometimes die and will be replaced with scar tissue. This is unsightly, and I see some of these patients on occasion. It is very difficult to explain that the smoking habit they have had for years is the cause, not necessarily a lack of skill on the surgeon's part.

As a patient, you must be open and honest with your surgeon. Most of the time, the doctor will ask you to stop smoking at least two weeks prior to surgery and for six to eight weeks after. The surgeon will warn you of the consequences and possible complications and keep a keen eye out for problems.

Alcohol and Recreational Drug Use

Surgeons are not the police or the moral majority, nor do they want to be. They are concerned with your health and your surgical outcome and, as such, need to be aware of your drinking habits as well as any drugs you might be taking. This includes prescription medication as well as recreational drugs.

Your doctor may ask you to stop drinking before and for several weeks after the surgery because alcohol can interact with drugs your surgeon may prescribe after surgery, specifically painkillers. Alcohol use, especially prolonged, can weaken the liver, which will be put under stress during your operation.

Prescription drugs can have many interactions and side effects, so a full disclosure of all the medication you have been taking is crucial. Medications such as anti-inflammatory drugs, which are often prescribed for arthritis, can lead to excessive bleeding. Your primary care physician can assist you in safely eliminating these drugs before and after your procedure until it is once again safe to take them.

Some common over-the-counter drugs are to be avoided as well. Aspirin and ibuprofen open up the blood vessels and can lead to excessive bleeding just like some prescriptions can. I always tell my patients to put these medications in a different location than normal before they come for their procedures. It is very easy after surgery to reach for the bottle of ibuprofen before you even think about it. It's habit for most people to take these medications when they don't feel well. Placing them somewhere else forces you to stop and think and helps keep you from making a mistake.

Likewise, many people regularly take herbal supplements. Many prescription medications are derived from herbs that can be bought in their diluted form over the counter. It is important to remember that, just like prescriptions, these herbs can have tremendous effects on the ability of the body to heal and to clot blood after surgery. Just to be safe, remove these from your diet for two weeks prior and four to six weeks after surgery.

High Blood Pressure and Heart Disease

Most patients with high blood pressure can safely have cosmetic procedures, provided that the blood pressure is well controlled. If not, it can cause additional bleeding after surgery, even to the point of needing a blood transfusion.

Many patients with heart disease, or even those who have had previous heart attacks, can have a successful cosmetic procedure as well. Just be aware that additional precautions will need to be taken. Your plastic surgeon may request a copy of your EKG from your cardiologist or ask that a current one be performed. Often, the plastic surgeon will ask that you obtain clearance from your cardiologist confirming the stability of your heart disease. There is no reason to become upset or alarmed at this. If your heart disease is unstable, putting you under anesthesia can trigger an erratic heart- beat (arrhythmia) or even cause a heart attack. Any plastic surgeon that requires these additional tests and clearances is only looking out for your safety.

Obesity

As I stated earlier, plastic surgery is no substitute for taking care of yourself, which includes eating right and watching your weight. Just because liposuction is available it is not a weight-loss option and shouldn't be considered as such. Liposuction and other body contouring procedures are designed to help you achieve a good result in areas that you otherwise couldn't. For example, you may have excess skin on or around your breasts, a wrinkled abdomen after having a baby, or small pockets of fat that just won't go away. No amount of exercise will ever correct these problems. And while plastic surgery can help with these problems, you have to know that it is not a quick fix, nor is surgery a replacement for a healthy lifestyle.

NOW IS THE TIME TO START IF YOU HAVEN'T ALREADY.

Excessive weight can also lead to breathing problems, which can be life threatening if the obese person is put under anesthesia. You have probably seen on TV that it is sometimes medically necessary to remove large sections of skin and fat to allow a morbidly obese patient freedom of movement so they can exercise. This is incredibly dangerous and potentially life threatening. Most of the time, this type of procedure is only performed when the patient's risk of impending death outweighs the life-threatening risk of surgery. This is inappropriate for most people. You must commit to a healthy lifestyle well in advance of any procedure. You want to take great care of your new body once you have it, and now is the time to start if you haven't already.

The most important thing to remember is that no matter what medical issues you have, you must talk openly and honestly with your surgeon. He or she will be able to provide advice and direction on how to cope with your specific problems and help you to achieve your best result.

NOTES

_____

_____

_____

_____

_____

_____

_____

_____

_____

_____

_____

_____

_____

_____

_____

_____

_____

_____

_____

_____

_____

_____

_____

_____

_____

_____

_____

_____

_____

NOTES

_____
_____
_____
_____
_____
_____
_____
_____
_____
_____
_____
_____
_____
_____
_____
_____
_____
_____
_____
_____
_____
_____
_____
_____
_____
_____
_____
_____
_____

NOTES

_____

_____

_____

_____

_____

_____

_____

_____

_____

_____

_____

_____

_____

_____

_____

_____

_____

_____

_____

_____

_____

_____

_____

_____

_____

_____

_____

_____

_____

_____

"AFTER THIRTY, A
BODY HAS A MIND
OF ITS OWN."
— BETTE MIDLER

CHAPTER 4
Body Sculpting for Men

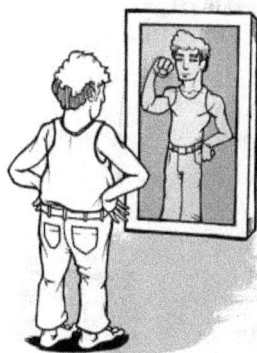

"The pain passes, but the beauty remains."

— *Pierre-Auguste Renoir*

Men are affected by the media's idealized version of beauty just as women are. The reasons behind a man's decision to have cosmetic surgery run the gamut from the desire for career advancement to simply wanting to feel better about himself.

As a man ages, he may feel the pressure of not looking as young as he used to look. This is especially true if the individual is in a position where he meets a lot of people and must look his best. Men identify very heavily with their profession, and the fear of being replaced by a younger version of yourself is very real. Also, the aging process isn't any kinder or easier to handle just because you are male.

I have seen a large increase in men opting for procedures including face-lifts, liposuction, and breast reductions. Men who have gained and lost a great deal of weight face some of the same issues as women, namely, eliminating loose skin. Fortunately, there are procedures that can have an equally fabulous result.

Gynecomastia

I see many men in my office who are concerned about the increase in fatty tissue and breast tissue in their chests. This is called Gynecomastia. The word Gynecomastia comes from the Greek word meaning "woman's breast." This condition can be very disheartening and psychologically devastating to men of all ages. Although in ninety percent of adolescent boys, symptoms of Gynecomastia (increased fatty tissue) will disappear, ten percent continue to have increased breast tissue, which causes psychological damage and physical shame. It is estimated by the American Society of Plastic Surgeons that Gynecomastia will affect an estimated forty to sixty percent of men. It can affect one or both breasts.

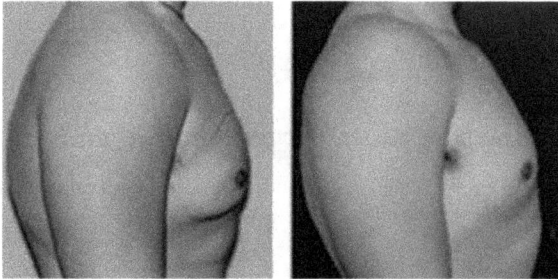

Preoperatively, patient had significant amounts of glandular and fatty tissue, requiring both liposuction and removal of gynecomastic tissue through a periareolar incision. Final results show tightening of the skin as well as flattening of the chest.

As you can imagine, men with this problem feel embarrassed and endure self-imposed exiles from any activity that might require them to take off their shirts. They are also limited in the types of clothing they will wear and are hesitant to be socially active. They see this condition as a loss of masculinity, and it can lead to depression and loss of self-confidence.

Certain drugs, including steroids and marijuana, and medical problems have also been linked to increased breast tissue. Psychologically, this can be a humiliating, devastating, and very embarrassing condition for men of all ages. The bottom line is that it makes a man feel less masculine.

The best candidates for Gynecomastic surgery are healthy males who have good elasticity of the skin. The patient should always refrain from drinking heavy amounts of alcohol and from smoking marijuana. Patients should also refrain from using any form of anabolic steroids at any time.

When a patient comes to my office for this type of procedure, I will usually ask that they see an endocrinologist prior to surgery. We need to determine if they have any form of hormonal imbalance, such as increased estrogen, within their blood. If this is the case, we must address this underlying medical issue prior to proceeding.

There are multiple approaches for Gynecomastic surgery. In the mildest approach, direct liposuction of the chest can be performed under general anesthesia. This will allow fatty tissue to be removed. If, however, there is also a significant amount of glandular and/or fatty tissue behind the areola, this generally can not be removed by liposuction alone, and often the patient will undergo a direct extraction of this glandular tissue through an incision underneath the nipple. This procedure is usually referred to as a partial subcutaneous mastectomy.

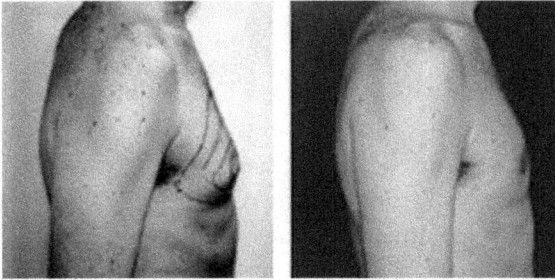

Patient had significant amounts of glandular and fatty tissue requiring both direct excision, as well as liposuction of the chest.

In the most extreme forms of gynecomastia, where there is also a significant amount of loose skin, the patient may actually undergo a form of breast reduction operation. It is a very similar operation to what I perform on women. It does leave an anchor-like scar straight down the middle of the breast and along the crease, but this kind of incision has to be done in order to allow removal of excess skin as well as glandular and fatty tissue.

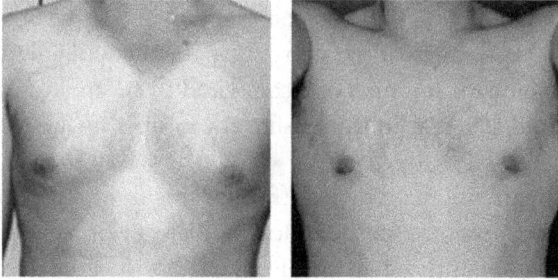

Patient underwent direct liposuctioning of the chest area with tumescent technique as well as direct excision of subcutaneous tissue through a periareolar approach. Patient has an excellent result.

Normally, patients remain in compressive garments for six to eight weeks after surgery to decrease the swelling. Sutures are most often removed by the 14th day after surgery, and all patients are told to refrain from heavy lifting for three to four weeks postoperatively.

In general, patients undergoing surgery for Gynecomastia are extremely happy with the results. Not only does it physically remove the often- painful glandular tissue, but it makes them feel better about their bodies and they get a tremendous psychological boost.

Liposuction for Men

Many men come to our office for a liposuction procedure, but unlike women, who may wish to have the procedure performed on almost any part of their bodies; the majority of the men desire to have liposuction in one area: their abdomen. The majority of the men I see for this procedure are unhappy because they have the "old spare tire around the belly." This means that they have some lower abdominal protrusion and fat that has concentrated itself in this one area. Many of them also have fat along the iliac crest rolls of the hip areas (love handles), it's that lower bulge that usually extends from hip to hip.

As we discussed previously, the patient must be a good candidate for the procedure and in relatively good overall health. During the initial examination, it is extremely important to differentiate whether the fat is outside the abdominal muscle or whether it is within the abdominal cavity (intraperitoneal), "the old beer belly." We cannot remove fat that is inside the abdominal cavity.

If a patient has a significant abdominal protuberance (a large abdominal girth), that individual is never a candidate for liposuction. He actually may not have enough fat for liposuction whatsoever or show any significant result from a liposuction procedure.

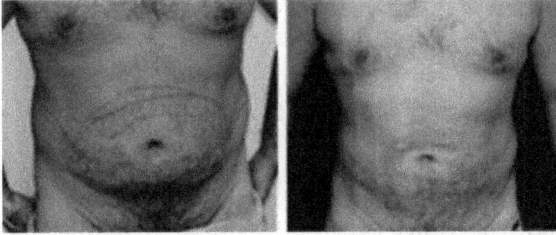

Patient underwent 1.8 liter tumescent liposuction in order to regain a better shape with localized deep fat removed from the abdomen and hip rolls.

After a clinical examination by the plastic surgeon, the doctor will easily be able to differentiate whether the fat is intraperitoneal (around the gut), or extra muscular fat that can be suctioned and will allow for a good result. Liposuction in men can also be a little more difficult than in women, because sometimes the fat is more dense, fibrous, and adherent to the layer over the muscle. It may not suction out as softly and smoothly. Male fat is more resistant and harder to extract; therefore, not as much fat is normally removed from men as is in women.

Women tend to have more of a spongy fat. When performing liposuction, this kind of fat tends to suction out easier and with less work on the surgeon's part. Thigh liposuction can also be performed on men, though it is very rarely seen in my practice. Most of my male patients come in for liposuction, almost exclusively, of the belly and occasionally for love handles.

The additional fat on men's hips can upset them just as it does women, affecting whether they can wear their jeans in a normal fashion, etc. Liposuction in men should be performed under general anesthesia administered by a board-certified anesthesiologist in a certified surgery center.

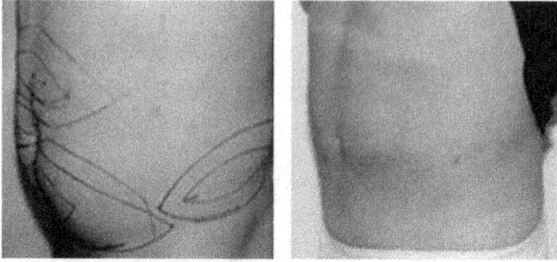

Patient underwent 1.5 liter tumescent liposuctioning of the upper and lower abdomen and hips. A signifigant change in appearance was achieved.

While it may seem that more is better, the amount of fat removed should be restricted. I like to extract no more than three to three and one-half liters per procedure. I tell my patients that they can stage the surgery. If more liposuction is required, we will wait four to six months and then undergo a second stage liposuction in order to prevent undue amounts of blood loss, which can be very dangerous.

It has taken a number of years for men to feel more comfortable with the idea of plastic surgery, though some still struggle with it. I would encourage any man to seriously weigh the benefits of plastic surgery, especially if he is living a self-imposed social exile due to body confidence issues. There is no need to ostracize yourself or feel the least bit hesitant about a procedure that will open new doors and generate a renewed feeling of self-worth.

NOTES

_____

_____

_____

_____

_____

_____

_____

_____

_____

_____

_____

_____

_____

_____

_____

_____

_____

_____

_____

_____

_____

_____

_____

_____

_____

_____

_____

_____

_____

_____

NOTES

_____

_____

_____

_____

_____

_____

_____

_____

_____

_____

_____

_____

_____

_____

_____

_____

_____

_____

_____

_____

_____

_____

_____

_____

_____

_____

_____

_____

NOTES

_____
_____
_____
_____
_____
_____
_____
_____
_____
_____
_____
_____
_____
_____
_____
_____
_____
_____
_____
_____
_____
_____
_____
_____
_____
_____
_____
_____
_____
_____

"PLASTIC SURGEONS
ARE ALWAYS MAKING
MOUNTAINS OUT OF
MOLEHILLS."
– DOLLY PARTON

CHAPTER 5
Breast Augmentation

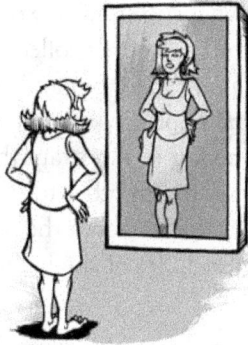

"The trouble with plastic surgery is that after 10 years gravity wins out and you have to have another one in about a year or so."

– Linda Evans

One of the most common procedures that women request in my practice is breast augmentation. For many women, breasts are an indication of femininity, and having very small breasts, or almost none at all, can impact the way a woman feels about herself. It also limits the types and variety of clothing she can wear. In today's body-conscious world, it can also be difficult to find clothing that fits correctly or looks good if her breasts are proportionally small.

Once you have made the decision to have your breast augmented, it is time to safeguard yourself. Breast augmentation can be very costly if done incorrectly. It is vital that you have realistic expectations and that you review many, many pictures of your doctor's work, both from a frontal view and the oblique or side view. The reason you must see the post-operation photos from the frontal view is that, sometimes an oblique or side view can be misleading. It is essential to look for symmetry of the inframammary folds which can only be visualized by the frontal view. If you see anything in these photos that concerns you, now is the time to discuss those matters with your doctor.

As you might imagine, implant size is a very important decision. Discuss with your doctor what cup size you would like to be and why. If there are some photos in the doctor's collection that are similar to the result that you desire, point these out and come to an agreement with your doctor on the size implant you want. Once the size of the implant has been determined, it is important that you understand the technique the doctor will use in order to place the implant. It is vital that you talk with your doctor about the safety issues involved in the technique and the reason he or she is choosing that particular technique.

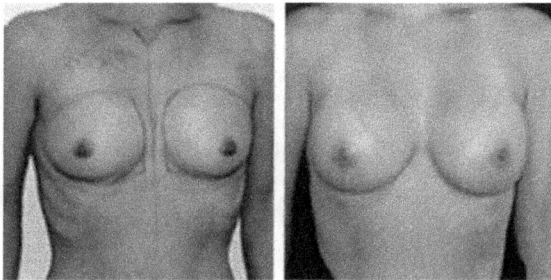

Preoperatively, patient was a 32A. 425 cc high profile smooth round saline implants were placed under the muscle with the incisions underneath the areola.

I prefer to use the periareolar approach when I do a breast augmentation. This approach is performed with an incision made underneath the areola. This, in my opinion, is the safest and most predictable approach. It allows the most accurate placement of either a saline or silicone implant under the muscle.

When placing the implant I also use the subpectoral, or "dual plane," technique. Instead of placing the implant either entirely under the muscle or entirely on top of the muscle, this is a hybrid type of placement. The first half to two-thirds of the implant is placed under the muscle on the side of the breast that is closest to your breast bone. The remaining third of the implant is covered by glandular material and left on top of the muscle.

This technique accomplishes several goals. By placing the inner portion under the muscle, it prevents the edges of the bag from showing in your cleavage area. This gives a very natural-looking result. Leaving the remaining third above the muscle allows for a round, youthful appearance to the breast when viewed from the side. This technique may also reduce scar tissue formation or capsular contracture, which is the hardening of your breasts. This technique is also more useful for accurate mammography in the future and may allow for an easier detection of small types of breast cancers.

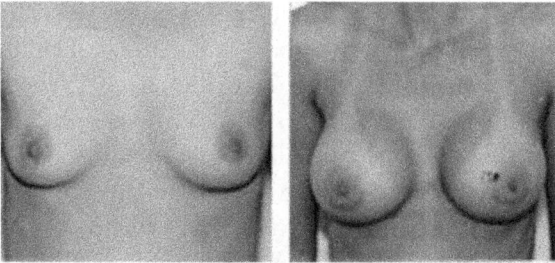

Preoperatively, patient was a full 32A. Patient underwent an augmentation mammoplasty procedure with 390 cc moderate profile smooth round saline implants placed through incisions underneath the areola in the dual plane technique.

Once you have decided to proceed with the operation, a preoperative visit is the next step. This is scheduled on a different date than the original consultation in order to discuss the following topics once again with the surgeon directly: the size of the bag, the shape of bag, the surgical approach, and postoperative management.

During your consultation with your board-certified plastic surgeon, one of the most important discussions you will have concerns the correct amount of fluid and/or the specific size of the prosthetic implant bag. These implants come in different sizes that are incrementally graduated, for example, 320, 350, 400, 425, 465, and so forth. The experienced surgeon will look at your anatomy and take into account your thickness of muscle, height, weight, and body frame, as well as your personality and social background. He will also consider your occupation to help make a decision regarding the final volume of your implants.

Remember, the stronger you are and the thicker your muscles in your chest, the larger the saline implant will need to be to overcome those muscles and give you more fullness. For example, if you're five feet even, weigh 145 pounds, and have a very strong upper build, this is referred to as an endomorphic body. You will be strong and may have a barrel chest, where there is very thick breast tissue and thick muscle, so your implant will need to be of a substantially large size in order to overcome the effects of that muscle and/or breast tissue and give you a good result. This is not unusual with very thick barrel-chested women, especially those of Latin descent. The implants may also have to be placed in a subglandular or retromammary pocket to allow for any fullness of the upper part of the breast. If an implant is placed behind the muscle in a very thick-chested woman with large amounts of both glandular breast tissue as well as muscle, the implant will be flattened and the woman will have a very unhappy final result.

One of my favorite questions to ask patients in consultation is this: "Which is worse in your opinion, to be slightly too large or slightly too small?" This is an extremely important question. If your answer is that it would be worse to be slightly too small (and that seems to be the most common answer), then consider going one implant size larger. For example, if you chose a 425 high-profile saline implant, but you're thick-chested with a wide chest diameter, you may want to go up to 465 high profile to give yourself a little more projection. You may also want to give the surgeon some leeway to overfill it if necessary, to give you that beautiful final shape. Always take into consideration that your anatomy is totally different from that of any other woman, and you can never compare your breasts with those of your girlfriend, mother, or anyone else. Since he or she will be better informed about your expectations, your doctor will make the correct decision with your help and your detailed instruction as to what you are looking for. The more pictures you review with the doctor, the better off you're going to be.

Be patient after this type of surgery and wait for the entire healing process to complete before making a judgment on your final result. Don't be alarmed that you overdid it. Your breasts will be swollen, and it will take some time for this swelling to dissipate.

Some of the issues that we try to impress upon our patients during the postoperative visit are things that they can do to reduce postoperative bleeding or a possible hematoma (collection of blood in the tissues). We stress not only that the patient not take any aspirin or aspirin-type products, such as Advil, Motrin, Excedrin, or Ibuprofen, that will thin the blood and cause more bleeding, but also that the patient should not do any heavy lifting. While most people begin to feel better a short time after surgery, we stress that the patient refrain from lifting for a full three to four weeks after surgery. Excessive lifting or straining may tear the muscle or cause an artery or vein to open, resulting in a hematoma or collection of blood, which may require additional surgery to repair.

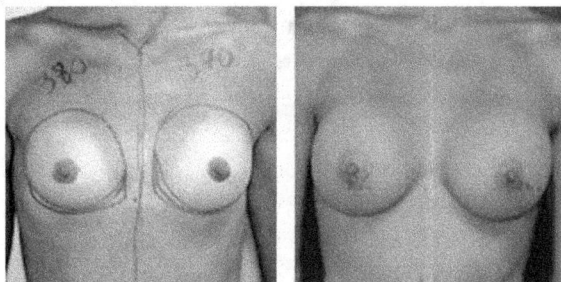

Patient underwent an augmentation mammoplasty procedure, a 380 cc high profile saline implant was placed on the right and a 370 cc high profile saline implant was placed on the left. The incisions are well-healed and the patient has an excellent and natural result.

We also stress that you refrain from smoking for at least two weeks prior to surgery and two months after, and cease the use of all alcoholic beverages. This will help the blood flow and promote healing, while decreasing the risk of drug interactions. These rules have greatly reduced our incidence of bleeding and infection, the two most common complications of any surgical procedure.

Another way we try to reduce the incidence of infection is to give our patients intravenous antibiotics approximately thirty minutes prior to surgery. We then place the patient under general anesthesia with a laryngeal mask airway, known as a LMA, by a board-certified anesthesiologist. General anesthesia puts the patient completely to sleep, you will have no feeling or remembrance of pain, nor memory of any part of the operation.

APPROXIMATELY NINETY PERCENT OF THE SWELLING WILL TAKE SIX TO EIGHT WEEKS TO RESOLVE.

After performing over 4,000 general anesthetics with the same anesthesiologist our office has not experienced any patient that has had any recollection or pain from the operation performed.

Once the procedure is complete, you will be cared for in a recovery room and will recover for a minimum of one hour to allow the anesthesia to wear off enough for you to awaken. Once discharged from the surgery center, you will be sent home or, if you have made prior arrangements, to a recovery hotel with well-trained registered nurses to care for you.

It is mandatory that you see the doctor the next day, at which time all dressings will be removed and compression garments (sports bras, abdominal binders, girdles) will be placed. After seven days you will see the doctor again, at which time an examination of the breasts will be conducted to make sure there is no evidence of infection or bleeding. Subsequent follow-up visits are generally scheduled at one-week intervals starting on day fourteen, when the sutures are removed from underneath the skin. Usually patients are told to take a sponge bath to reduce the chance waterborne infections until the sutures have been removed. Our patients are also placed on one week of postoperative antibiotics, as well as pain management with codeine products such as Vicodin or Darvocet in order to reduce immediate postoperative pain.

When I perform this procedure I use a subcuticular closure, meaning the sutures are placed under the skin. This technique helps reduce scarring. Normally the incision sites are cleared of sutures by day seventeen and patients then can resume taking showers or baths.

Approximately ninety percent of the swelling will take six to eight weeks to resolve. You should consult with your doctor immediately if you have increased swelling, fever, or increased pain or redness of the breasts at any time. Successful breast augmentation surgery requires not only an excellent and experienced board-certified plastic surgeon who specializes in breast enhancement surgery, but also a well-informed patient who will conform to and obey the rules that are given by the surgeon. When the patient has followed the surgeons orders they can expect a successful recovery.

SARAH'S STORY

Sarah is a twenty-two- year old, Caucasian female who came to see me because she was unhappy about the size of her breasts. She is approximately 5'2" and weighs 121 pounds. When I examined her, I found that she had minimal to no breast tissue and was a 32AA. Sarah's complaint was she was unable to wear formals, lingerie, or bikinis during the summer months with confidence. She wanted to look and feel better, after a bit of discussion, Sarah decided that she wanted to be proportionate for her frame, thereby, a mid-C cup. We talked about the technique that would be used, as well as all of the safety factors of which she needed to be aware.

Sarah was in overall good health and decided to proceed with breast augmentation surgery. We had a long discussion about avoiding all alcohol and aspirin products both before and after the surgery. We also talked about things she could do to ensure a speedy recovery.

> HER BREASTS LOOKED PERFECT AND SHE WAS VERY HAPPY WITH THE RESULTS.

On the day of the procedure, Sarah went to the operating room, was put under general anesthesia, and had an excellent and uneventful operation that lasted less than one hour. She did not experience any post-operative bleeding or significant pain.

In the recovery room, ice compresses were placed on her breasts and she was sleeping in an elevated position in order to reduce swelling. An hour later, she was awake, given her discharge instructions and once again reminded not to do any form of lifting for the next few weeks and to keep her incisions dry for the next fourteen days. The next day, during her follow-up, Sarah had her dressings removed and was placed in a sports bra with an upper pole compression strap at the top, which would allow the implants to settle into the perfect position over time. I reminded Sarah to continue to take the prescribed antibiotic and to take the pain medication only if she was having pain. Sarah was advised that taking pain medicine unnecessarily could cause the following symptoms: nausea, vomiting, and possible constipation.

One week later, she came in to see me again for a quick visit, just to make sure that there were no signs of infection or bleeding and that the implants were settling in the appropriate positions. Dressings were now being changed twice a day, and she returned seven days later, on day fourteen, and her sutures were removed. She was delighted with her appearance. She had nice C cup breasts. The swelling was resolving nicely as well. At that time she was instructed that after seventy-two hours, she could take her first shower, but she should still refrain from pools, sauna baths, or any submersion in water for another three to four weeks. Her breasts looked perfect and she was very happy with the results.

Sarah was seen again four weeks later, at which time her incisions were fully healed. She could now start working out and was starting to do some mild tissue expansion or massaging of her breasts to soften the pockets, and she could now wear a regular bra. Sarah was very happy and, soon after, brought her girlfriend in for a consultation for the same procedure.

Silicone versus Saline: What's New

During your consultation, questions will arise as to which implants are best for you. Should you use silicone or saline? As of November 17, 2006, the FDA has approved silicone implantation once again. This is an amazing result after fourteen years of struggling with the manufacturers to prove that there is no causal relationship with autoimmunes disease or cancer when a patient has silicone gel implants. At the present time, breast augmentation with silicone implants may be performed on women who are at least twenty-two years of age, for both primary breast augmentation as well as for revision breast surgery. As in the past, Silicone implants may be used for patients who undergo breast reconstruction for any form of breast cancer or trauma surgery.

THE FDA HAS APPROVED SILICONE IMPLANTATION ONCE AGAIN.

When women consider silicone gel augmentation, many factors need to be reviewed and discussed prior to having surgery. You should first determine whether silicone gel or saline is right for you. This is a patient specific question, and each woman needs to understand that her body is different, just because your girlfriend has silicone implants does not mean that this is the best choice for you. When considering silicone gel implants it is very important to understand all of the safety issues.

There are several factors that should be taken into account when determining if silicone gel implants are right for you. Anyone with active infections in their bodies, existing cancer or pre-cancerous conditions, and those who are presently nursing or pregnant should not use silicone gel implants. Women with autoimmune diseases, a weakened immune system, or who have had radiation to their breasts following breast cancer should be cautious when choosing silicone gel implants. Patients who have experienced poor wound healing in the past should also be cautious. Psychological issues may also preclude the use of silicone gel implants in women; these issues would include depression or other like symptoms.

EACH WOMAN NEEDS TO UNDERSTAND THAT HER BODY IS DIFFERENT.

Capsular contracture (scar tissue forming around implant) is also quite high with silicone implants and is more common in secondary or revision augmentations than in primary. This means that if you have had your breasts augmented and you are going to have a revision surgery to remove scar tissue, your chances of more scar tissue reoccurring is higher the second time around, according to studies conducted by Mentor Corporation. Capsular contracture will also increase your risk for implant rupture. Capsular contracture can occur either with silicone or saline implants and may require removal or release of the scar tissue around the implant.

With silicone, fifteen percent of women who have undergone primary breast augmentations will have re-operation within the three years. Twenty eight percent of women who have had breast revision surgery using silicone implants will have a third surgery within the following three years.

While you must understand these facts, silicone implants are still wonderful products and many women feel they are softer and look and feel more natural than saline. Patients also like the fact that there is less visibility of the implant bags.

When implants are placed in thinner women who have less breast tissue and thinner muscles, silicone gives a better result, at least early on, because there is less rippling and visibility of the implant bag. On the other hand, a woman who has a very thick chest and large amounts of glandular breast tissue as well as very strong muscles, will usually do better with saline implants and have fewer risks and problems associated with scar tissue or rupture. Because silicone implants look and feel so natural, they have become an implant of choice for many women. Just remember, silicone implants have a significantly higher rate of scar tissue formation and hardening around the bag. The chances of having multiple surgeries with silicone implants are great.

Silicone implants can rupture or leak and may require replacement. It may be more difficult to detect a rupture with silicone because often it will go undetected, unlike those with saline, where, if they rupture, the implant completely deflates and the breast with the ruptured implant becomes significantly smaller than the opposite side.

When you're considering silicone gel implants, it is very important to realize that implants are not life-time devices. Per Mentor Corporation's description, "breast augmentation is not a one-time surgery." Implants often need to be removed and replaced throughout a woman's life, and with some women many times.

It is also very important to understand with silicone implants that implant ruptures are often "silent." Silent means that neither the woman nor the surgeon may even know that it is ruptured, and only an MRI can determine whether it is truly ruptured. According to Mentor Corporation, one of the world's largest leading silicone implant manufacturers with FDA-approved implants, the ability to determine a rupture on physical examination by a Board Certified Plastic Surgeon is approximately 30% versus 80% with an MRI. Therefore, with the FDA approval of silicone gel implants physicians are now recommending that women with these implants have an MRI three years after surgery and then again every two years after that. It is also important to realize that MRIs are extremely expensive and some healthcare insurers do not cover them. Your potential rupture rates with silicone implants, according to Mentor's core studies, are approximately .5% through three years for primary augmentations (1 out of 200 patients) versus 7.7% on MRI over a three-year period for patients who have had revision augmentations. In other words, your rate of rupture is much higher in patients who are having secondary surgery.

Mammography is an X-ray exam of the breast. This exam is extremely important for detecting and evaluating the breast for any type of abnormalities. Doctors recommend mammograms both for screening purposes, when patients have no symptoms or complaints, and diagnostic purposes, when patients do have symptoms or complaints. These symptoms can include a lump, discharge from the nipple, or increased pain localized along the breast.

Routine screening mammography can be more difficult with silicone implants. Silicone gel implants may make it harder to visualize small malignancies than saline. Also, additional x-ray views are required on patients with silicone implants versus saline, which may increase the women's exposure to radiation. Some patients may be surprised to find their health insurance premiums may increase, or they may be dropped completely, if they choose silicone implants. It is very important that you investigate and analyze these possibilities with your health insurance carrier prior to making your decision to determine the specifics of their coverage with silicone implants.

THE INCIDENCE OF BREAST CANCER IN THE UNITED STATES RANGES FROM NINE TO ELEVEN PERCENT OF ALL WOMEN, AS REPORTED BY MANY DIFFERENT STUDIES FROM THE AMERICAN CANCER SOCIETY.

According to the Centers for Disease Control (CDC), from 1999 to 2002, over 182,000 new breast cancer patients were diagnosed. Mammography has proven to be the best way to find cancer of the breast, from its earliest stages, up to three years before a woman can actually feel a lump. The mammogram can also locate small cancers that are too fine to be felt or noticed during a clinical breast examination.

Remember that your risk for breast cancer will increase greatly as you age. Screening mammography should normally be done on a patient every year beginning at age forty. Patients with implants should have a mammography performed every year after the age of thirty-five. This could reduce mortality by twenty to twenty-five percent over ten years for women over the age of forty who have mammograms every year. Facts about breast cancer can be found through the National Breast Cancer Awareness website. There are predisposing factors for breast cancer, and we will take some time to talk about a few of these.

First, tumors need to be differentiated between cancerous or malignant tumors, and benign, not malignant or non-cancerous tumors. In order for a cancer to be malignant, it simply means that the cells are growing uncontrollably, they become invading and they damage the surrounding tissues. This can then lead to the cells metastasizing, spreading into the blood or the lymphatic system. The incidence of breast cancer in the United States ranges from nine to eleven percent of all women, as reported by many different studies from the American Cancer Society.

Increased breast-cancer risk factors include

1. **Age.** The older a woman is, especially once over age 60, the greater the risks for breast cancer.

2. **Race.** Some studies have shown that African American women may have an increased risk over women of other ethnic backgrounds.

3. **Family history.** Family history of breast cancer is a strong indicator of increased risk. If your mother, sister, or daughter has breast cancer, there is an increased, and more significant chance that you may as well.

4. **Personal history.** If you have had a history of breast cancer, there is a greater risk that you may develop it again. There are breast cancer genes that have been shown to increase the risk of cancer as well.

5. **Estrogen.** Estrogen is a hormone that occurs in every woman, but at increased levels it may also increase your risk of breast cancer. Increased estrogen situations can include a) having your first period at an early age, before the age of twelve; b) a pregnancy occurring at a later age, after the age of thirty-five; c) having no children, as women who have never been pregnant have increased levels of estrogen throughout their lives; d) taking hormonal replacement therapy; and e) taking oral contraceptives.

6. **Lifestyle changes.** These may also increase and/or reduce your risk of cancer. Decreasing your fat intake, increasing your fiber, limiting alcohol, reducing smoking, and staying active can all significantly reduce your risk of cancers of the breasts.

MAMMOGRAPHY IS MORE DIFFICULT IN YOUNGER WOMEN, SINCE THEY HAVE MORE DENSE FIBROUS TISSUE

The American Cancer Society recommends screening for breast cancer at an early age. Women in their twenties and thirties should have clinical breast exams by their professional healthcare provider at least every three years. After age forty, clinical breast exams should be performed every year with mammography. Detection of breast cancer is normally performed with the aid of diagnostic mammograms. These often require magnified views to see lesions that could not be seen on the original. Normally, a mammography will take about twenty minutes, with results available within thirty days Statistics have shown that two to four mammograms out of every 1,000 will lead to a diagnosis of cancer. Ten percent of woman who have mammograms will require another test; usually additional mammography imaging, ultrasound, or a breast biopsy is required.

Surgical biopsies are often performed in order to determine specific details of something that was seen on the mammogram. These biopsies can include wire localization, in which the mass is localized with a small wire and samples of cells are removed, or a needle biopsy, which involves a fine needle or a larger core needle to directly excise the complete lesions through an external approach. Biopsies are usually done by a general surgeon.

Interestingly, mammography is more difficult in younger women, since they have more dense fibrous tissue, which can make it more difficult to visualize tumors. It is not uncommon that a breast ultrasound will be done as well as a mammogram in order to properly screen women who have extremely dense breast tissue. Ultrasounds may also be useful in determining suspicious areas, such as a cyst, or may be useful for guiding the needle biopsies. MRIs can be used for patients who have very dense breasts. They are also very useful for patients who may have ruptured silicone gel implants. The FDA feels that only the MRI is useful for determining whether a silicone gel implant has been ruptured.

Breast Augmentation

The Eklund technique has been devised for performing mammography on women with breast implants. This technique is called the "displacement view." Extra views and time are needed for this; therefore, patients should tell the scheduler prior to the appointment that they have breast implants, so extra time will be allotted. The displacement procedure normally involves pushing the implant back and pulling tissue into the view so that it can be compressed and mammograms can then be taken. Sometimes it is more difficult to perform the Eklund technique in women who have severe scar tissue or capsular contracture and women who have very dense or fibrous breasts. Implants placed above the muscle can also make it more difficult to determine microcalcifications. Scar tissue around the capsule can be difficult to differentiate from calcification, which could be associated with cancer and thereby require an actual biopsy.

It is extremely important to have a mammogram performed at the correct time. If a patient has a family history of breast cancer and is going to undergo elective breast augmentation, I believe that she should have a mammogram and possibly an ultrasound as well, which will provide the surgeon with a road map. Normally, a woman would not need to have her first mammogram before the age of forty, however, I prefer to have my patients get a baseline mammogram prior to surgery regardless of age.

In my practice, I have found that there is also increased scar tissue formation with silicone rather than saline implants. This may be associated with the silicone gel bleed. In other words, the oil from the silicone migrates through the small micropores and through the shell of the bag. It then gets trapped around the scar tissue that forms around the implant. A mammography can be more difficult to read due to interference associated with silicone implants, as they may hide or mask small calcifications or even small cancers.

The patient should also be concerned with possible migration, where the silicone can bleed out of the shell of the implant and actually migrate to the lymph nodes, the glands underneath the armpits, and possibly to other parts of the body. Because of all these issues, patients must think very carefully about whether they really want to have silicone implants put into their bodies.

Post-operatively, you must also remember that if you are having dental work you must take preventative antibiotics prior to your dental procedure.

In general, saline implants seem to have fewer risks associated with them. With saline implants, we are able to change fill volumes of the bags; this offers more flexibility for women who have significant asymmetry. You can adjust the volumes to even out the breasts and make them more symmetrical. Though saline implants may rupture, the patient will know within a few weeks that her implant is deflated. Fluid from a saline implant is quite safe. It is usually normal saline solution, which will be absorbed into the body, and the patient will just eliminate it through natural body functions. Should this happen to you, it is important to have the implant replaced sooner, rather than later. The longer you wait the greater your chance for additional scar tissue forming around the bag, requiring surgical intervention to restore a normal appearance to that breast.

COMMONLY ASKED QUESTIONS DURING CONSULTATION

1. **What size implants should I consider for my body type and frame?**

   This is very personal and probably one of the most important questions that a patient who is considering having breast augmentation surgery will ever ask. The patient needs to take many factors into account; the first one being overall build, or height and weight. The proportions of a woman's body are extremely important. As a plastic surgeon specializing in body work, I look at every single patient as a unique individual. Just because your girlfriend Mary has full C cup breasts and went with a 500 cc implant, there is absolutely no reason for you to do the same. If your body is different in size, shape, height, and weight, then a different size implant will probably be suggested to give you the result that is right for you.

For example, if a woman is 5'7", is a 32A, and has a moderate build (not too thin, with some significant body fat and breast tissue with thick pectoralis muscles because she works out hard), she may want to be a full C and, therefore, possibly somewhere between a 450 cc and a 490 cc round saline implant will be used. If, on the other hand, the woman is very petite (thin and has a very minimal amount of breast tissue and very thin muscle), is five feet even, and is a 32AA, she may only want a 350 cc round, smooth saline implant that may be filled to 370 cc to give her between a mid and full C, which would then be proportionate for her size.

Implants should always be tailored to the patient. Each woman is so totally unique that a doctor must make the beauty of the implant match the woman's physique.

2. How much cleavage will I have?

Cleavage really depends upon several factors. The first factor is the distance between a woman's breast folds (intersternal distance).

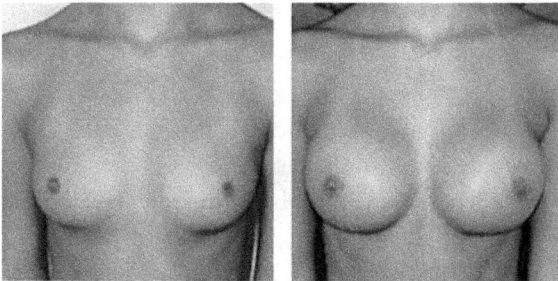

Cleavage was obtained by placing 400 cc high profile saline implants behind the muscle in the dual plane and releasing the inner aspects of the pectoralis muscle and limiting the outer pocket dissection.

The further apart they are, the further the muscle is inserting into the ribcage or along the sternal border and the further the muscle attaches to the chest wall, up and down or side to side, the less cleavage the woman is going to have. It is very important that board-certified plastic surgeons not completely release the muscle when we dissect underneath it. This allows for good coverage of the implant along the middle of your chest, and helps prevent rippling and/or visibility of the implant bag.

3. How wide of an implant should I get?

The wider the implant, the more cleavage the woman will probably have if a pocket is made correctly and not open too far on the side.

4. How concerned should I be with the technical ability of the surgeon?

You should be very concerned and aware of the technical abilities of any surgeon. The implant pocket has to perfectly fit the implant. If a pocket is made larger than the implant the implant may slide to the side causing the patient to have no cleavage, mis-shaped breasts and the appearance that the breasts are flopping to one side.

5. How much recuperation time will I need?

This is an excellent question that is specifically determined by the type of work that a woman does. In my practice, women who work in an administrative setting or women who work in an environment where they don't have to do heavy, labor-intensive lifting usually require five days off work before they can return. Patients whose jobs are more labor-intensive, such as, anyone who uses their upper body, shoulders, arms and hands, will greatly increase their risk for bleeding and tearing of the muscles if they start back to work too early. They may require up to three to four weeks off of work to allow for safe healing.

6. **When will I be able to shower or bathe?**

In my practice, patients are instructed not to get any form of water on or near the incision site for fourteen days. They may sponge bathe immediately. The incision sites must remain clean and dry to reduce any type of infection, including staphylococcus or streptococcus skin infections.

7. **Where are we going to place the implant, above the muscle or below the muscle?**

This is a pretty easy question. I believe that the majority of breast augmentations should be performed with the implant placed using the dual plane technique. This means that the middle half of the implant is placed under the pectoralis muscle and the lateral half or lateral third is placed under the glandular tissue. There are several advantages to this approach of placing at least half of the implant medially under the muscle. First, you reduce visibility of the implant bag and it is not felt along the midline or along the middle of the chest. Second, you reduce the incidence of scar tissue, which is a hardening of the implants that has been shown to be much worse when the implants are placed above the muscle. Placing the implants under the muscle may lubricate and allow the implants to remain softer. Third, this approach allows for better mammography. It has been shown mammography is easier for the radiologist to interpret when the implants are placed under the muscle. This is especially important if the patient has a family history of breast cancer. Finally, this approach allows for a more natural appearance. Placing the implants under the muscle leaves less rounding along the upper portion of the breast, which may look fake and unnatural.

8. **Should I limit my chest building exercises after I am healed from my breast augmentation surgery?**

I feel that once a patient has had implants, she should refrain from doing extensive chest building exercises again. Unless she is a professional athlete or fitness champion in competition, working out the or the chest muscle causes thickening and flattening of the implant and actually makes the implants look less full and less attractive. So, the vehement answer is, the patient should never extensively exercise her pectoralis major muscles again after subpectoral augmentation surgery.

9. **Is it true that I may get stretch marks after I have surgery?**

It is absolutely true. The larger the patient decides to go, the greater the chance that stretch marks may occur. Stretch marks occur with small scars and cracks in the skin surface, especially with a very large expansion or stretching effect. For example, if a woman has a 32AA and goes to a full C, the chances of developing stretch marks are very significant. The stretch marks will often appear very red and will radiate from the areola like sun rays. They will, thankfully, fade with time, and the small capillaries and small blood vessels will turn white and appear much less obvious. You may decide to use topical solutions both before and/or after surgery on your breasts to help reduce this effect. Vitamin E and Palmer's Cocoa Butter have shown to be useful with our patients.

THE TEN BIGGEST MYTHS ABOUT BREAST AUGMENTATION

Myth #1: Breast Implants Can Cause Cancer

False: Studies or experimental data have not been able to link breast implants with cancer.

Myth #2: Breast Implants Must Be Removed Every 10 Years

False: There is no specific data on duration of time for implant replacement. The implants may last a lifetime or only a few years, depending on complications, including deflation, scar tissue formation, or choice to change the size of the implants.

Myth #3: I Should Never Wear an Underwire Bra with Implants

False: Underwire bras can and should be worn, but only once all healing has occurred. Over time, without proper support, the weight of the implants can create significant sagginess and stretching of the breast tissue and skin, which an underwire bra can help prevent.

Myth #4: Shaped Implants Are More Natural Than Round Implants

False: Imaging studies of the chest have shown that both shaped (anatomical) and round implants appear to have a similar natural slope when properly placed under the muscle. One complication of shaped implants is rotation of the bag, which can lead to disfigurement.

Myth #5: Loss of Sensitivity of the Nipple Is Associated Only with the Periareolar Approach

False: Numbness can occur from any approach if the nerves are stretched or traumatized during surgery.

Myth #6: Mammograms Are Not Possible with Implants

False: Placement of the implants, either silicone or saline, under the muscle will help with Displacement Technique Mammography and allows for excellent mammography results.

Myth #7: Women over the Age of 50 Should Not Undergo Breast Augmentation

False: Patients of any age may undergo the implant surgery as long as they are healthy, in good medical condition, and free of breast cancer. Lab work is required for all surgical candidates, and a routine mammogram is required for anyone over the age of thirty-five or with a family history of breast cancer.

Myth #8: The Most Common Reason for Reopening the Incision Is the Patient's Desire to Remove the Implant Entirely

False: Actually, deflation (eighteen percent) and capsular contracture (eighteen percent) are the top two reasons for reopening or undergoing a second procedure.

Myth #9: More Women Desire to Go Larger on the Next Surgery and Believe That They Went Too Small Originally

True: Women become accustomed to the swelling that generally occurs during the first two to three months after surgery. When that subsides, they miss the fuller feeling and desire to have slightly larger implants put in to compensate for the loss of the swelling.

Myth #10: It is easy to detect a rupture or tear in a silicone gel implant.

False: Silicone ruptures are often "silent" because the implant holds its shape and may go undetected for years. An MRI is the most definitive method for determining a rupture or tear.

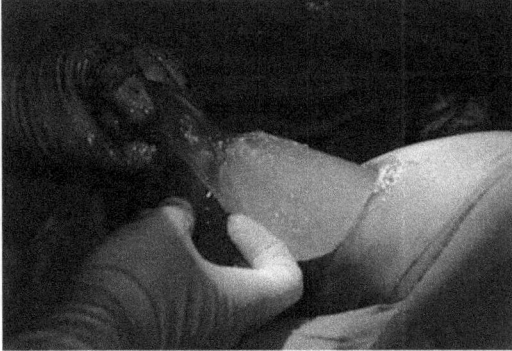

Interestingly, mammograms were negative and patient was referred to Dr. Linder by a different surgeon. Dr. Linder's revision of this patient included removal of silicone gel implant material, removal of scar tissue and capsule, lowering of the implant pocket and replacing with new cohesive silicone gel implants.

NOTES

_____

_____

_____

_____

_____

_____

_____

_____

_____

_____

_____

_____

_____

_____

_____

_____

_____

_____

_____

_____

_____

_____

_____

_____

_____

_____

_____

_____

_____

NOTES

_____

_____

_____

_____

_____

_____

_____

_____

_____

_____

_____

_____

_____

_____

_____

_____

_____

_____

_____

_____

_____

_____

_____

_____

_____

_____

_____

_____

_____

_____

_____

_____

"Pain is inevitable.
Suffering is
optional."
– M. Kathleen Casey

CHAPTER 6

Breast Revision, Correcting Surgery Gone Wrong

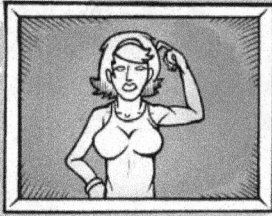

"Sex appeal is fifty percent what you've got and fifty percent what people think you've got."

— *Sophia Loren*

Many women have undergone breast augmentation surgery and are extremely happy with their results. Not only does it enhance their self-esteem but also makes them feel better in and out of clothes. Unfortunately, there are also a significant number of women who are not satisfied with their results.

The first thing that I want to impress upon you is having realistic expectations. You have to ask yourself if your results fall within the reasonable category based upon on where you started. If you are feeling unsure about your surgical outcome, ask your surgeon for your before pictures and compare them to your result. It is sometimes difficult to remember how far you've come and easy to focus on very minor imperfections. I suggest that you step back and get a true perspective of your individual situation.

The second area I find many patients dissatisfied with is the healing process. Don't be impatient; some individual patients bounce right back, and some don't. Give your body time to heal. It may take six months just for the swelling to completely go down, and scars will fade over time. Be gentle with yourself during this time. Rushing into another surgery to fix or repair something is not a good idea when you haven't given your body time to readjust and heal properly.

YOUR DOCTOR'S FIRST CONCERN IS ALWAYS TO ACHIEVE THE BEST RESULT POSSIBLE WITHOUT DOING ANY HARM.

The last area of concern for many patients has to do with the final results. In previous chapters you read about the differences in each person and how specific medical conditions can affect your surgical outcome. It is important to remember this when assessing your results. Did you follow your doctor's instructions after surgery? Do you have one of the known risk factors that can affect healing after surgery? Discuss these with your doctor, and let him know how you are feeling. He can help alleviate any concerns you may have or follow you more closely if it appears there is a problem.

Let's assume that you have honestly considered all of the above areas and you are still dissatisfied with your results. The first course of action is to discuss the issue openly with your doctor. If you are still unhappy, then you should seek a second opinion. Be sure you choose the same level of board-certified plastic surgeon as you did the first time. You must be aware that this surgeon may agree with your first doctor and tell you that your results are within the normal expectation range.

Your doctor's first concern is always to achieve the best result possible without doing any harm. When a surgeon thinks about revision of a previous surgery, the risk of making matters worse has to be weighed against the possible outcome. To be honest, sometimes it is just not worth it, but as the patient, this can be difficult to hear. Please try to maintain as much objectivity as possible before considering another surgery.

NECESSARY REVISIONS: CAUSES AND CURES

True dissatisfaction from breast augmentation surgery can occur for many reasons. One of the most common is that the patient may have had implants that were either too large or too small. The patient may have gone to a doctor who was not qualified to do the surgery, which may significantly increase the risk of having an unacceptable final result.

On the other hand, the patient may have simply developed numerous problems resulting from natural body changes and medical conditions that occur over time.

The most common natural phenomenon causing patients to return to our office is scar tissue formation with hardening of the breasts, referred to as capsular contracture. The body forms it's own protective barrier surrounding any type of surgical material or implant placed. The body creates a barrier of collagen, fibroblast and blood vessels to protect itself. These form a glistening white capsule around the implant bag.

This is completely normal. In the event the bag should tighten and harden, or become visibly distorted, this can be extremely painful and is referred to as a Baker IV Contracture. Inamed Corporation has shown that up to sixteen percent of women will develop severe encapsulation of their breast implants approximately seven years after surgery. Correction will include either removing the capsule, a procedure called a capsulectomy, or releasing the capsule, a procedure called a capsulotomy.

When a woman has had multiple surgeries on her breasts or has very thin breast tissue, we don't like to take out much scar tissue because this will thin out the tissue covering the implant and make the bag more visible. Seeing an implant bag through the skin is distressing.

Another common reason for revision surgery is that the initial implant was placed improperly. I see this on a weekly basis with patients who have their breast implants placed through the navel (transumbilical) or under the armpit (transaxillary approach). Let's face it, inserting an implant through the belly button and tunneling all the way under the muscles to the breast seems like an awfully long distance. In actuality, it is, and results from these procedures can be very unpredictable. While patients sometimes ask for these types of approaches because they leave no scars on the breast itself, I still don't believe that it is a good trade-off if you end up unhappy and deformed.

One of the most disturbing malformations after surgery occurs when the implants are placed too high and create a what is known as a double-bubble deformity.

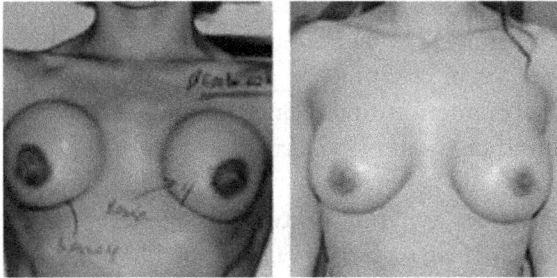

Severe scar tissue, capsular contracture with painful breast deformity. Patient required bilateral release and removal of scar tissue and replacement with 390 cc saline implants.

This happens when a surgeon places the implant in an improper position and the skin overhangs the implant and looks like two different breasts flopped over each other. I see these quite often. These cases are very difficult to rectify, but I am able to fix them in most cases.

JACQUELINE'S STORY

Jacqueline came into my office approximately eight months after undergoing her breast augmentation with a different surgeon. During our initial consultation, she expressed that she was extremely unhappy with the appearance of her breasts.

As we discussed the details of her first surgery, it became clear that she did not realize that she went to a non-board-certified plastic surgeon. In fact she didn't even go to a plastic surgeon at all. The doctor who performed her breast augmentation surgery was a dermatologist. This doctor did not have the training, experience or qualifications to perform breast augmentation surgery, and unfortunately, Jacqueline was now suffering the consequences.

She felt that her breasts were totally deformed, and I had to agree. Her right breast had the classic double-bubble appearance, as her implant was placed way up under her clavicle, leaving the skin to hang loose at the bottom of her breasts. Jacqueline had previously breast-fed two children and her breasts already were quite saggy. She'd also had natural loss of volume. She truly needed a formal breast lift. Instead, she now had the implant in the wrong position and the skin overhanging her breast.

This can be very difficult to remedy, but she made the correct decision to have this corrected by a qualified plastic surgeon with the training to accomplish the task. Jacqueline and I talked at length about how to repair her botched surgery. I advised her that in order to achieve the best results, the implants would need to be removed and replaced with high-profile saline implants.

SHE WAS EXTREMELY HAPPY WITH THE APPEARANCE OF HER BREASTS.

The scar tissue would be released, and the new implants placed in the proper position in the pockets. I would then perform a formal breast lift, which should have been done from the beginning.

Remember, if you go to a doctor and his solution to your problem sounds too good to be true, such as, "Oh, you don't need a breast lift," when you really feel in your heart and your mind that you do, you will probably be disappointed. Like Jacqueline, you will need to visiting another surgeon's office to have this surgery corrected.

Jacqueline agreed with me that she wanted the best results possible and underwent the removal of scar tissue, replacement of the implant bags, lowering of the implants, and corrective breast lift surgery. Three months after the surgery she was extremely happy with the appearance of her breasts. Once her incision healed she started using Mederma scar cream three times daily and Vitamin E on the incision sites; this helped to smooth and fade the scars. Her scars looked good, but there was a little redness around the incision sites that will continue to fade over time.

Jacqueline had been instructed to perform regular massaging of her breasts, to wear regular bras, and always to wear a sports bra at night in order keep the implants in the proper position. This patient's experience is a good example of the pain and suffering that can occur with an unqualified doctor.

Pregnancy, Breast-Feeding, and Ruptures

Once a patient has had breast augmentation, she must understand that future pregnancies and breast-feeding may cause dramatic changes. These might include changes to the pocket that holds the implant and increased scar tissue formation around the implant bag, causing major distortions. It is important to plan for this and be aware that if you choose to have children after surgery, you may also be looking at revision surgery of some kind down the road.

Then there is, of course, the threat of rupture. One of the questions I hear most often is, "Can these implants rupture, and if that happens, what do I do?" The majority of the implants we use are saline implants, which means they are filled with a salt and water solution. If they were placed under sterile conditions and filled with sterile fluid, then the body will absorb the fluid and there should not be any complications. However, you will want to have that implant replaced as quickly as possible. The longer you wait, the lower the likelihood of a good result as scar tissue can form after the collapse. Implants can rupture at any time, so understand that this is a real possibility. The two major manufacturers of implants in the United States both have lifetime guarantees on replacement of the implant bags.

OTHER ISSUES

There are several other issues that we see on occasion. While not as common as the ones listed above, they do occur.

Bottoming Out

"Bottoming out" simply means that there is sagging of the skin, and the implant falls with gravity, making the breast look very odd. The nipple ends up on top of the breast, and the implant ends up very, very low. The implant will typically slide down along the chest wall.

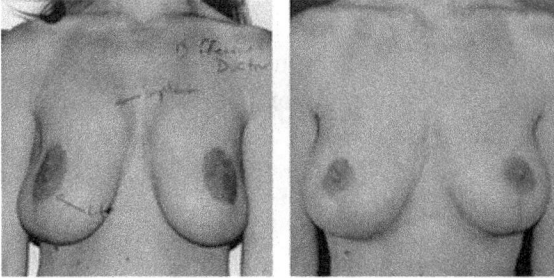

Original surgery performed by a different surgeon. Implants were placed in the improper position and caused bottoming out of her breasts as well as widespread scarring and enlargement of the areolas. Patient underwent removal and replacement of the implants with a smaller size implant, as well as a revision breast lift and areolar reduction.

Fortunately, this is not very common. We have had to correct a lot of these due to the use of less predictable placement techniques, such as the trans-auxillary (under the armpit) or trans-umbilical (through the belly button) approach.

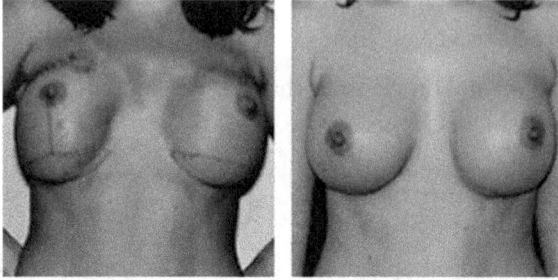

Original surgery performed by a different doctor. Revision included removal and replacement of saline implants, removal and release of all scar tissue, internal capsulorrhaphy, tightening of the internal capsule as well as an inframammary breast lift (removing redundant excess skin along the inframammary fold). Patient has an excellent result.

To correct "bottoming out", you may require a procedure called a capsulorrhaphy or tightening up of the internal capsule. In this instance a breast lift may be required, which will leave external scarring, and may potentially require placement of a smaller implant.

High-Riding Implants

In the case of "high-riding" implants, the doctor positions the implants in too high. The most common cause of this problem is when the muscle is not accurately released along the sternum or the lower fold during surgery. The implants don't fall into the correct position and are therefore too high. This may result in the patient looking like she has a more masculine chest. As you can imagine, most patients are very dissatisfied with this result and unhappy with their appearance.

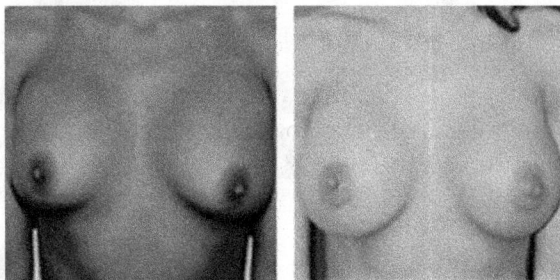

Patient had severe encapsulation and scar tissue around both implants. The implants were positioned superiorly with a very unnatural appearance and painful breast deformity. Surgery included release and removal of the scar tissue (open capsulotomy) and replacement with 510 cc saline implants.

This is another example of why not to use the trans-axillary (under the arm) or the trans-umbilical (through the belly button) approach. The results of improper placements from these approaches can leave patients very dissatisfied with the outcome, requiring a second or even a third surgery. The operation necessary to correct this problem will involve releasing and lowering the fold to allow the implant to fall into a natural position.

Anatomical Implants

Due to the many complications associated with Anatomical or Tear Drop implants, I do not recommend nor use them in my practice. The largest risk being rotational deformity, which means that the implant bag flips around. Even a five degree turn will cause the breast to look completely deformed. The odds of it reoccuring and requiring revision after revision make it not worth it.

BREAST AUGMENTATION SURGERY WORKSHEET

Prior to your surgery there are a number of items that you **must** discuss with your doctor. I have provided the following worksheet to help guide you through this process. You should bring a copy with you to each consultation.

APPROACH OF PROCEDURE

Where will the incisions be made?

> Periareolar
> Trans-Umbilical
> Trans-axillary
> Other _____

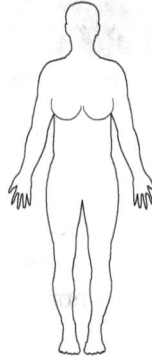

Where will the implant be placed?

> Behind the Muscle
> Above the Muscle

What kind of implant will be used?

> Saline
> Silicone
> Other _____

What size of implant will be used?

> _____ cc
> Filled to? _____ cc
> Manufacturer? Inamed, Mentor or other _____

Will a concurrent breast lift be performed?

_____

If so, what type? _____
Periareolar, vertical, or anchor scar

What are the credentials of the anesthesiologist?

Are they board certified? Yes or No

What is the accreditation of the ambulatory surgical center?

_____

Be sure to carefully review all consent forms and documentation.

Additional Questions

_____

_____

POST-OPERATIVE WORKSHEET

Be sure to keep your post-operative instructions and paperwork for future reference. This can be very instrumental in the event you require revision surgery at a later date. This information will allow your doctor to understand your prior surgery so that you may receive optimal treatment.

Items you keep on file:

Implant manufacturer _____

Implant information

Serial #   _____
Lot #   _____
Catalog #   _____
Size   _____

Name of plastic surgeon   _____
Date of surgery   _____
Location of Surgery   _____
Were biopsies performed? Yes or No
If yes, be sure to retain a copy of your pathology report

Also be sure to obtain a copy of your operative report.

DATE AND TIMES OF FOLLOW-UP APPOINTMENTS

Month	Day	Time
_____	_____	_____
_____	_____	_____
_____	_____	_____
_____	_____	_____
_____	_____	_____

NOTES

NOTES

_____
_____
_____
_____
_____
_____
_____
_____
_____
_____
_____
_____
_____
_____
_____
_____
_____
_____
_____
_____
_____
_____
_____
_____
_____

NOTES

_____
_____
_____
_____
_____
_____
_____
_____
_____
_____
_____
_____
_____
_____
_____
_____
_____
_____
_____
_____
_____
_____
_____
_____
_____
_____
_____
_____
_____
_____

"FALSIES ARE THE
BUST THAT MONEY
CAN BUY."
– BOB LEVINSON

CHAPTER 7
Breast Reduction

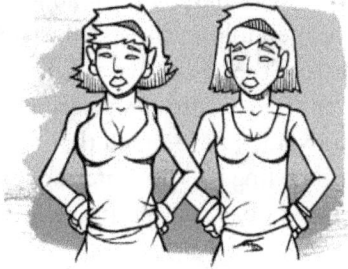

"I'm tired of all this nonsense about beauty being only skin deep.
That's deep enough. What do you want, an adorable pancreas?"

— Jean Kerr

Though many women long for larger breasts and a more
proportional appearance, there are a small number who have
exactly the opposite problem. Women of all ages come to my office
every week requesting that I reduce the size of their breasts. These
women do not have breasts that are merely larger than the average
woman's, their breasts are enormous. This can cause a myriad of
health problems, including extreme back and neck pain, shoulder
deformation, and rashes that often turn into fungal infections of
the skin.

During pregnancy, some women develop gigantic breasts that never
return to normal, the most common cause of this problem is genetics.
At times, I will see several members of the same family, mothers and
daughters who have inherited this problem and have passed it on.

I hear from women of all ages about the terrible symptoms they are experiencing due to their massive breasts. Bilateral breast hypertrophy/gigantomastia is simply breasts that are way too large for a woman's proportion.

No woman should have to live her life in constant pain from the size of her breasts or endure any of these symptoms. The patients I see are experiencing most, if not all, of the following symptoms:

1. **Back Pain** – These women have not just above-average sized breasts, but gigantic, pendulous breasts. Most patients endure chronic back pain from the additional weight they carry. Many begin to hunch over and have trouble maintaining a normal posture. Numerous women have stated that they feel as if they are carrying enormous bowling balls or watermelons with them 24 hours a day. This type of back pain is unrelenting.

2. **Rashes** – Many women with large sized breasts experience frequent skin rashes, especially during the summer months. These rashes can develop into infections that have an unpleasant odor associated with them. This can become an extremely embarrassing hygienic problem.

3. **Shoulder deformation** – Over time, women with very large breasts will develop deep grooves in their shoulders. They're painful and can cause scarring of the shoulder blade area. This stems from the weight of their breasts, which causes the straps of their bras to dig in.

4. **Neck pain and headaches** – Due to the weight on the chest, neck pain, headaches, and upper back pain are common complaints also. While many patients who suffer with this condition use over-the-counter medications, sometimes for years, to ease their symptoms. They soon discover that there is no topical solution and that their pain only gets worse with time.

5. **Inability to wear normal clothing** – Most of these patients body type does not allow them to buy clothes off the rack in most department stores. Many find that they must order their clothing from specialty companies or have them handmade. They also have trouble finding a large enough or properly fitting bra in any conventional store. Many of these women have bra sizes that escalate into the EE, GG, HH, and II categories.

6. **Psychological embarrassment** – People often gawk and stare at women with large breasts, and many find that they attract unwanted attention wherever they go, making them very self-conscious. Some become introverted, refusing to go out in public due to their appearance and often hide under baggy clothing.

Now that we have discussed the problem, let's talk about what can be done to alleviate it. In general, women considering this procedure should be very healthy. Nonsmokers are preferred, since smoking inhibits the healing process and increases the risk of skin loss due to lack of blood supply and increases the possible death of tissue around the nipple areolar complex. Though it is rare, the odds of this complication happening can be lessened by choosing a board-certified plastic surgeon who specializes in this procedure.

BREAST REDUCTION IS A MAJOR SURGERY THAT REQUIRES PRECISE SKILLS BY THE PLASTIC SURGEON.

Any patient considering a breast reduction should also be cleared by a general internist and her family practitioner, who will certify her overall medical health. If you have hypertension, diabetes, or other medical conditions, those need to be well controlled prior to undergoing this operation.

It is important to understand that a breast reduction is a major surgery that requires precise skills by the plastic surgeon. The most common and most conventional technique used to perform this procedure is referred to as the anchor scar technique (Wise-pattern technique).

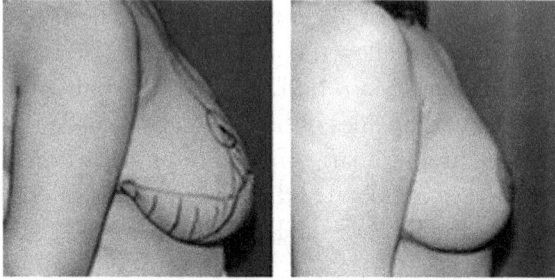

Severe bilateral breast hypertrophy. Patient's symptoms included back pain, neck strain and grooving along her shoulder blades. Patient underwent a breast reduction using the Wise-pattern inferior pedicle technique.

This technique allows the tissue to be removed from the inner and the outer aspects of the breast as well as above the nipple. It is performed by removing skin, fat and glandular tissue in all three quadrants, allowing the breast to be made significantly smaller, and it raises the nipple up to a more Natural position. The skill level of this surgery is greatly advanced due to the fact that the blood supply within a woman's breast area is very vulnerable. The doctor must be well versed in the surgical dissection and make sure that the blood supply is maintained at all times.

The most satisfied patients of all, certainly in my practice, have been patients who have undergone a breast reduction procedure. These results have been backed up by data from the American Society of Plastic Surgeons as well. Not only does a breast reduction alleviate all the symptoms described above, but it helps women feel better about themselves by giving a more normal appearance to her breasts.

The way I perform a breast reduction procedure is similar to the way I perform a breast lift. The incision sites are fairly the same and produce an anchor-shaped scar consisting of a straight line from the bottom of the nipple extending down to the crease, followed by a semi-circular line in the crease.

The major difference, of course, is that during the breast lift surgery the surgeon usually isn't removing any breast tissue. They are just removing the skin. With a breast reduction, you are not only removing skin, but also fat and glandular tissue as well.

Breast Reduction

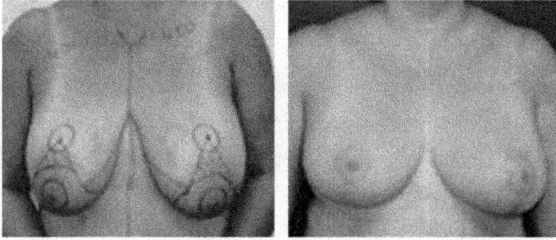

Patient had 38EEE breasts with severe sagginess. Symptoms included shoulder grooving, back pain, neck strain and rashes under her breasts. Patient underwent a breast reduction using the Wise-pattern technique. Over 500 grams were removed per breast.

All tissue removed is sent to pathology to screen for breast cancer. This is another reason to have a mammogram and/or ultrasound done prior to undergoing a breast reduction. It is very important to have a road map of your breasts prior to surgery, because all of the tissue becomes quite distorted after the doctor removes and repositions the different areas of the breasts.

A drainage tube will be in place for the first twenty-four to forty-eight hours to prevent excess fluid buildup. After the tube is removed, you will wear a sports bra for approximately three to four weeks to mold the breasts. Sutures may be left in from fourteen to twenty-one days, depending upon the healing process. Dressings will need to be changed daily. All patients are placed on antibiotics for one week and given pain medication, if necessary, for the first seven to ten days.

Without a doubt, incision sites and scars are your trade-off after breast reduction surgery. This is an operation in which there is a great deal of stress placed upon the incisions. Therefore, you may have very noticeable scars. If you are not willing or able to endure the scarring associated with this type of surgery, especially the anchor scars, then you may want to reconsider this type of surgery due to the likelihood that you will never be happy with the results.

One of the things I will stress concerning this procedure is that every patient must have realistic expectations.

MARY'S STORY

When twenty-two -year-old Mary came to my office, she was very distraught about her appearance. Her breasts were enormous, and while she had suffered emotionally for a number of years, the physical symptoms were now wreaking havoc on her life.

When I initially examined Mary she already had grooving in her shoulder blades that was cause scarring on her shoulders. She complained of pain of the upper and mid-chest areas as well as neck pain and chronic headaches due to the weight of her breasts.

Mary's 36EE breasts were also causing rashes and fungal infections under her breasts on and off over the past few years. Mary was desperate to have a breast reduction procedure to abate all of her symptoms. I discussed the procedure with Mary in detail.

> SHE IS DELIGHTED WITH THE APPEARANCE OF HER BREASTS AND NO LONGER FEELS THE SYMPTOMS OF BACK OR NECK PAIN

The next time I saw Mary was on the day of her surgery. At this time, I marked out the areas of tissue to be removed and the new position of the areola. I performed the operation, removing over 620 grams from her right breast and 640 grams from her left breast. Since her breasts were also asymmetrical, this corrected that asymmetry.

Small drainage tubes were placed in the breasts for one day and removed the next. Mary's surgery went well and was uneventful. The day after surgery, the nipple areolar complexes were pink and healthy, indicating that the blood supply was good and that healing would progress well. Mary was very happy.

Once the dressings and drains were removed, she was placed in a sports bra. Approximately fourteen days later, the sutures were partially removed. By day twenty-one, all of the stitches were taken out. Mary continued to wear a sports bra for approximately six weeks and now has full 36C breasts. She is delighted with the appearance of her breasts and no longer feels the symptoms of back or neck pain and all the grooving and rashes are gone. She feels good, she looks good, and her self-esteem has been immeasurably enhanced.

NOTES

NOTES

NOTES

"LOVE OF BEAUTY IS
TASTE. THE CREATION
OF BEAUTY IS ART."
– RALPH WALDO EMERSON

CHAPTER 8
Breast Lift

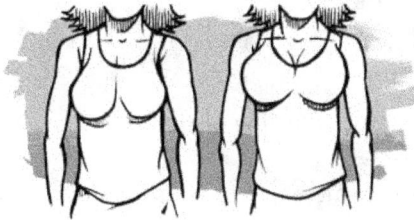

*"A beautiful thing never gives up so much
pain as does failing to hear and see it."*

— *Michelangelo*

We have discussed in the last few chapters that sometimes a breast lift is necessary to achieve a good result. But how do you know if you need a lift? Most women realize that their breasts won't look the same after they have children or if they lose a significant amount of weight. The skin of the breasts will stretch, and in this case, gravity affects their shape. As you age and experience a natural decrease in the volume of breast tissue, you will find that your breasts sag. It is as natural as it is inevitable.

Many women have thought about having this condition corrected but are nervous about the scars. Rumor has it that they can be pretty awful, and I can tell you that sometimes this is true. Since this is a procedure that involves removing excess skin, there is no way to prevent a scar.

In some cases, the scarring can be quite distressing, and I think it is important that we talk about this. You must consider what will be best for you and whether or not your expectations are realistic. The decision that you have to make is whether perkier breasts are a sufficient trade-off for scars that can be unpredictable.

In order to help you make that decision, let's discuss how scars work. Scarring is what occurs when the body heals an external incision site.

These scars can look:

- Great, hardly even visible
- Average, visible, but not bad
- Awful, to the point of feeling disfigured

Your scars, or lack thereof, will be the result of a combination of issues, including genetics, overall health, skin type, and skill of the surgeon. A bad result isn't necessarily the fault of the surgeon nor is it the fault of the patient. However, the skill of your surgeon and how you take care of yourself after surgery do play a significant part.

Let's start with the surgeon. Surgical technique is extremely important in regard to scarring. Board-certified plastic surgeons are well trained and qualified. They possess the skill to perform subcuticular closures in most circumstances. This means the sutures are placed underneath the skin, which will reduce the track marks that may occur when the sutures are placed externally (outside) and loop around the incision. Always ask your doctor how the suturing will be performed. With a breast lift, it should be done subcuticular. It has been my experience that this technique gives the best results.

Now, let's talk about the patient. Individuals don't heal the same. Remember when we talked about how your specific medical conditions, age, and stage of life affected your procedure? This is also true with scarring. You may have a girlfriend who had her breasts lifted and her scars are barely noticeable. On the other hand, her mother may have had the same procedure, and yet her scars extensive. Each person is different.

One important component to scarring is the amount of pigmentation and melanin in the skin. Ethnicity plays a large role in certain types of scars as well. In general, patients of Latin American, Korean, Japanese, African American, and Middle Eastern descent have more pigmentation and darkening of the skin, which may increase the risks of scarring. They may experience both darkening as well as keloid (raised scar) and/or hypertrophic scars.

It is an excellent idea to look at how scars have healed on other parts of your body, although this is not an absolute indication that incisions on the breast will heal exactly the same way. For example, if your C-section scar looks great, then it is easy to assume that your tummy-tuck or breast-lift scars will heal well, too. Although this is not one-hundred percent accurate. Because of the placement of the incision, there is very little tension on a C-section incision, which is usually why it heals nicely. However, the tension associated with the incision from a breast lift or tummy tuck can produce more extensive scarring.

THERE IS A PREDISPOSITION FOR KELOID AND HYPERTROPHIC SCARRING IN CERTAIN ETHNIC GROUPS.

When the doctor removes skin from the breast or the abdomen and pulls the edges of the wound together, the incisions can stretch, spread, and thicken as they heal. So, having a good scar in the C-section area does not mean that your scars from these other operations will be perfect or even the same.

I mentioned earlier that there is a predisposition for keloid and hypertrophic scarring in certain ethnic groups. It is more prevalent in African American and Middle Eastern populations, and it can run in families. This is a very important consideration when deciding to have a surgery such as a mastopexy or breast lift, where scarring can be significant.

CANDIDATES FOR BREAST LIFTS

Candidates for breast lifts usually include women who have a severe amount of sagginess to their breasts. This usually will include those individuals whose nipples are located below the inframammary fold. The inframammary fold is the crease under the breast and is the demarcation line when the doctor determines the degree of sagginess, (referred to as ptosis in Latin). Where the nipple lies in relation to the inframammary fold gives us the degree of ptosis. Very severe ptosis, with the position of the nipple well below the fold, indicates a need for a breast lift in which skin is removed both underneath the areola and along the fold.

This is what results in the anchor scar that we have discussed previously. In a breast lift, the incision goes around the areola, down in a straight line from the areola to the inframammary fold and then in a semicircular line along the fold. This technique allows us to limit the amount of skin removal, and to hide some of the incision underneath the breast crease.

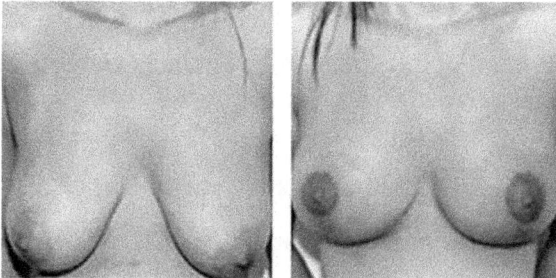

Patient is a 22-year-old Korean female presenting with severe grade III ptosis. The nipple areolar complexes were well over 3 cm below the inframammary fold. Patient underwent a formal mastopexy (breast lift) using the Wise-pattern technique. She is six months out and happy with the final outcome. Notice, no implants were required on this patient.

Another type of breast lift that is available is the periareolar or crescent lift, where a small amount of skin is removed from above the areola and the nipple complex is moved up. This is useful only in very, very mild cases of breast ptosis or sagginess. Often, this is combined with a breast implant placed under the muscle.

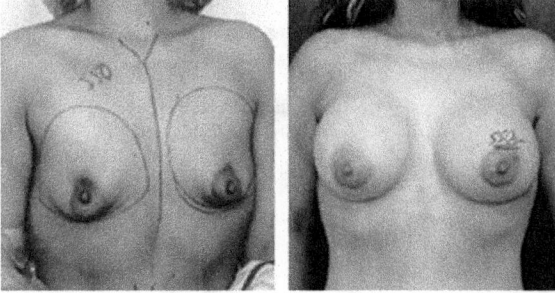

Patient required implants placed in the dual plane under the muscle, 550 cc saline implants were placed in order to regain fullness, as well as a periareolar crescent lift was performed on the right nipple in order to elevate it superiorly to match the left side.

Unfortunately, the results from this procedure are not very good. It does not address a truly severe amount of skin laxity. Some patients try this procedure in order to avoid a full breast lift, but they end up returning and having a total breast lift performed.

The next type of lift is referred to as the vertical lift. This involves removing skin in a donut fashion around the areola and lifting it below the areola in a vertical plane up and down. This will often allow for a nice tightening of a breast with moderate skin laxity. Often an implant is placed behind the muscle if the patient doesn't have enough breast tissue and/or volume.

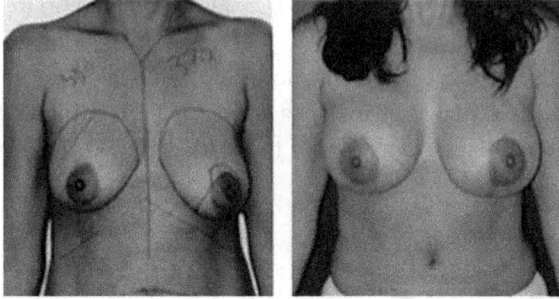

Patient underwent a vertical breast lift on the left breast in order to reposition the nipple at the same level as the right side. She also had implants placed to regain fullness of her breasts bilaterally.

The last type of breast lift is the full breast lift or formal mastopexy, which usually addresses the most severe form of ptosis, grade III, where there is a great deal of skin laxity involved. To correct this problem, we use the Wise-pattern or anchor-scar lift. This is usually going to produce the most beautifully shaped breast because it is really addressing all the problems of a sagging breast. These include too much skin below the areola in a vertical plane (up and down), as well as excess skin along the fold. I perform this procedure most of the time for severe skin laxity/looseness. When combined with implants in patients with loss of breast volume, especially after breast-feeding, this technique leads to beautifully shaped breasts.

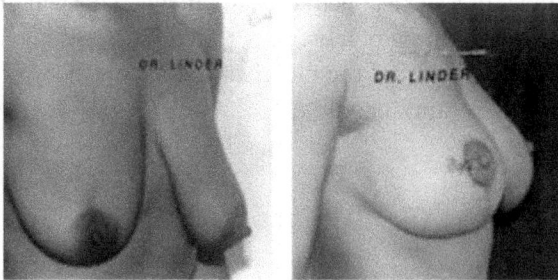

Patient had severe sagginess (grade III ptosis) with the nipple areolar complexes well below the inframammary fold. Patient underwent a formal mastopexy (breast lift) using the Wise-pattern technique, without glandular tissue removal, only skin was removed. Postoperatively, patient has a fantastic result.

Breast Lift

Prior to having a breast lift, I encourage patients to undergo a preoperative mammogram and/or ultrasound. As with a breast reduction, this will provide a baseline road map as to what the breasts looks like. We pay special attention to fibroadenomas (small little benign tumors) or cysts in the breasts, which can more easily be seen postoperatively or after your surgery. Any patient over the age of thirty-five should always have a mammogram and/or ultrasound prior to surgery, I can not stress this enough.

Patients often ask me about breastfeeding after a breast lift. Studies show that anywhere between five and fifteen percent of women will lose the ability to lactate or breast-feed following this procedure. This is a very important factor to consider when deciding to have this operation. No plastic surgeon can guarantee that you will have one-hundred percent sensitivity or the ability to breast-feed after a breast lift or breast reduction procedure.

MARIA'S STORY

Maria came to my office with very saggy breasts. Her breasts were large, and she was happy with the size but not the sagginess. Maria was forty years old, had three children, and had breast-fed all of them. Her breasts used to be perky but were now stretched out and unattractive. She was very unhappy with the changes in the appearance and shape of her breasts. She wanted to have them lifted. We discussed that the size of the breasts would go down almost one cup size after surgery due to the removal of excess skin. At our initial consult, Maria was a D cup. She stated that she would be happy to be a full C cup after the procedure. We agreed that no implant would be used, and she would simply have the formal mastopexy, removing the skin in the anchor-like pattern. The scars were a big trade-off, but she had realistic expectations of the outcome. After viewing thousands of photos, Maria decided the scars were worth the trade-off.

Maria's surgery went well, no complications, and she maintained sensitivity of the nipple areolar complex. In Maria's case, the nerves seemed to be well intact and she was delighted since there was a twenty-percent chance that she could have lost sensitivity to that area..

All of her stitches were removed by post-op day number seventeen, though she still remained in a sports bra for four weeks total. She now wears a regular bra and uses a scar cream three times a day. Maria is delighted and happy with the results, scars and all. She has been instructed to wear under wire bras the rest of her life, as well as sports bras while sleeping, in order to help maintain the lift of her breasts and prevent recurrent breast sagginess.

NOTES

_____

_____

_____

_____

_____

_____

_____

_____

_____

_____

_____

_____

_____

_____

_____

_____

_____

_____

_____

_____

_____

_____

_____

_____

_____

_____

_____

_____

_____

_____

_____

NOTES

_____

_____

_____

_____

_____

_____

_____

_____

_____

_____

_____

_____

_____

_____

_____

_____

_____

_____

_____

_____

_____

_____

_____

_____

_____

_____

_____

_____

_____

_____

_____

NOTES

_____

_____

_____

_____

_____

_____

_____

_____

_____

_____

_____

_____

_____

_____

_____

_____

_____

_____

_____

_____

_____

_____

_____

_____

_____

_____

_____

_____

_____

_____

"A THING OF BEAUTY
IS A JOY FOREVER."
– JOHN KEATS

CHAPTER 9

Abdominoplasty

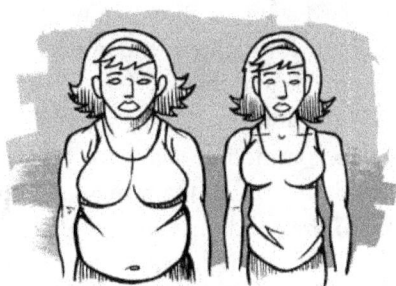

*"There is but one temple in the universe
and that is the body of man."*

– *Martha Graham (1894–1991)*

Abdominoplasty, more commonly known as a tummy tuck, is the removal of both skin and fat from the lower abdomen. The surgeon also tightens the internal muscles of the abdomen that run vertically from the ribs to the pubic bone. Occasionally, during a tummy tuck, the surgeon will also perform liposuction to the hip area in order to slim the entire midsection.

Tummy tucks are excellent procedures for the right kind of patient. One of the trade-offs, though, is a large scar that traverses the entire lower abdominal area. Normally, the scar is at about the same level as a C-section scar, but much longer, typically extending from hip to hip. The other incision made during this procedure is around the belly button. Given that a tummy tuck involves removing excess skin and tissue in the lower abdominal area, the skin from the upper abdomen is stretched down to close the wound. The surgeon must cut around the belly button and make a new hole for it further up on the abdomen to achieve a normal-looking result. The position of the belly button does not change along the abdominal wall, although the patient may feel that it was placed higher due to being accustomed to the excess skin pulling it lower on the abdominal wall.

The best candidates for tummy tucks are women who have already had all their children. As I stated earlier, in a normal tummy tuck, the surgeon tightens the muscles that run vertically in the abdomen.

LIPOSUCTION OF THE HIPS CAN GREATLY ADD TO A GOOD RESULT WITH A TUMMY TUCK.

Since pregnancy stretches these muscles to accommodate a growing baby, we often don't tighten them if a woman still intends to have more children. Otherwise, this area might pull apart during pregnancy once again.

While anyone over the age of eighteen can contemplate having a tummy tuck, they are most helpful to those who have had massive weight loss or have an increased amount of skin laxity due to multiple pregnancies. For women of childbearing age and intent, this procedure can be helpful and increase their self-esteem and body image. However, we don't tighten the muscles in these women, and they may not have as good of a result as they would otherwise. As long as the patient goes into the procedure fully aware that pregnancies can increase the odds of them needing a second tummy tuck, we can and will proceed.

Liposuction of the hips can greatly add to a good result with a tummy tuck. It may seem odd that your surgeon wants to address an area that does not bother you, but rest assured they are addressing this for a reason. Please be aware that changing one part or proportion of the body will enhance others, whether it be for better or worse. When a tummy tuck is performed and the hips are left as is, some patients complain that they feel broader than before, and the removal of the abdominal skin can result in them actually looking heavier on the sides. For this reason, I usually recommend suctioning the hips if there are significant amounts of fat in the hip regions. To me, it is very important to make the woman look narrower and thinner after a tummy tuck. That is why she is having the procedure done in the first place. She wants to feel better about her total midsection, not just her abdomen.

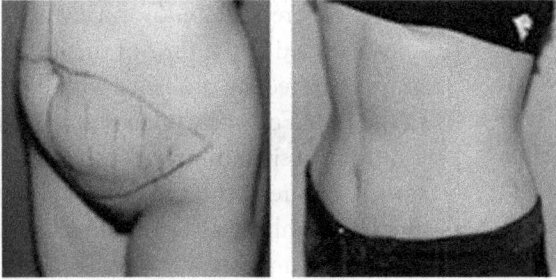

Patient underwent a tummy tuck (abdominoplasty), tightening of the muscles and removal of the redundant skin and fat. She has a well-healed scar which is hidden beneath her clothing.

Some patients come to my office complaining of laxity, or looseness, of the skin around the belly button. This is called mid-abdominal skin laxity. Usually in this situation there is not enough extra skin in the lower abdominal area for them to undergo a full tummy tuck. Just because you have loose skin on the abdomen doesn't mean you're a candidate for a tummy tuck.

In theory, in order to do a full tummy tuck, there should be enough loose skin so that it can stretch from just above the belly button all the way down to the incision above the pubic hairline. If there isn't enough skin and there's too much tension, it may be impossible to close the wound, and this could have disastrous results.

The decision on whether you have enough skin must be made by a qualified board-certified plastic surgeon. Again, the amount of skin and the location of that skin will determine whether or not you are a candidate for a full tummy tuck.

One of the things that surprise many patients is when their doctor suggests that the abdominal surgery be performed in two surgeries, rather than one. This is called staging and is very common in plastic surgery. Don't be surprised if your surgeon suggests this.

When a tummy tuck is staged in two surgeries, the first surgery may include removal of the skin and fat from the lower abdomen and liposuction of the hip area. The second surgery may include liposuction of the upper abdominal area above the belly button and below the ribs, as well as the sides of the abdomen above the hips (flank areas).

ALLOWING THIS FLUID TO DRAIN THROUGH THE TUBES SPEEDS THE RECOVERY PROCESS AND ADDS TO THE COMFORT LEVEL OF THE PATIENT.

These areas should normally not be liposuctioned at the time of the initial surgery in order to reduce problems with blood supply to the flap. For safety purposes, I also like to wait four to six months after the tummy tuck surgery before I sculpt the upper abdominal area. Remember, safety and predictability is of the utmost importance when considering any form of plastic surgery procedure, so if it takes a few months and a couple of surgeries to get the best result, then that is the path to take.

After your tummy tuck, you should expect to have drainage tubes. These may not be pleasant, but they are very necessary. After a large procedure like this, fluid may build up in the tissue, causing swelling. Allowing this fluid to drain through the tubes speeds the recovery process and adds to the comfort level of the patient. The tubes will remove fluid that is usually watery and reddish. You or your caregiver will empty the drainage every six hours. Once there is less than twenty-five cc's per day per tube, which is usually at least seven days, the tubes can be safely removed. Normally, they stay in place from seven to ten days.

There is a myth circulating through the rumor mill that pulling out the drain tubes is painful. It's not. Taking the drainage tubes out is a painless procedure performed in your surgeon's office, and it usually takes about two seconds per side. So if you've heard that this process is extremely painful, rest assured that it is not.

Abdominoplasty

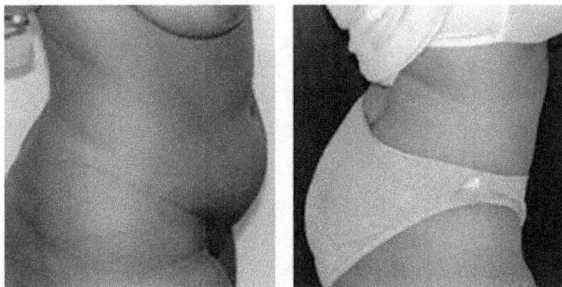

Patient underwent a tummy tuck (abdominoplasty) with skin and fat removed from the lower abdomen and tightening of the muscles. As well as liposuctioning of the hips to give patient a flattened stomach.

After a tummy tuck, I prefer to leave sutures in for fourteen to twenty-one days in order to prevent the incisions from opening up. The stress and tension placed on the incision site after this particular procedure is considerable, and I like to give the body additional time to secure the wound. Compression garments are also used after surgery for six to eight weeks. These help to compress the entire surgical area as well as the surrounding tissue. This facilitates the reduction of swelling.

Combination procedures can often be performed with tummy tucks. However, it is important that the doctor determine the amount of time under general anesthesia, as well as the possibility of blood loss and fluid shifts, when considering combining other procedures with tummy tucks. If the tummy tuck is a very large one, it may be a good idea not to combine a procedure like a breast augmentation or liposuction of the thighs with it. These are both major procedures with a potential for quite a bit of blood loss. For safety purposes, you may want to consider waiting three to five months or longer to allow the tummy tuck to fully heal before considering another procedure.

We have discussed scarring in relation to other procedures. For tummy tucks, scarring is a huge component. You must weigh very carefully your potential outcome against any scars that you might have. These scars are permanent and are never one-hundred percent predictable. There is always the potential for the scarring from this procedure to be quite unsightly.

PATIENTS WHO
HAVE REALISTIC
EXPECTATIONS
WILL GET
REASONABLE
RESULTS.

If you are not ready to accept scars and want a doctor to guarantee what your final scar will or will not look like, then you are not ready for this operation and should not undergo the surgery. Patients who have realistic expectations will get reasonable results and will be very happy afterwards. Those without them could, unfortunately, end up very depressed and wish they'd never had the surgery at all.

GLORIA'S STORY

Gloria had given birth to three children. She was in good shape and looked great-with her clothes on. With her clothes off, she had a tremendous amount of loose skin from the belly button all the way down to the pubic area. This excess skin bothered her a great deal. In fact, she was so self-conscious that she refused to wear a two-piece bathing suit.

Though only thirty-six years old, Gloria was certain that she was not having anymore children. She was ready for the full tummy tuck. After doing quite a bit of research on the Internet, Gloria was referred to me by two of her girlfriends. After examining Gloria's abdomen and talking to her about the results she wanted to achieve, I recommended a full tummy tuck. This meant removing skin from just above the belly button to just above the pubic hairline. Gloria also had a small bulging amount of fat on her hips. This would be sculpted and liposuctioned at the same time as her tummy tuck was performed, helping narrow her stomach area and her sides.

Gloria's surgery went well. Her drainage tubes were removed after one week, and she continued to wear a compression garment for about six weeks. Her stitches were totally removed on day fourteen. I also recommended that she start using a scar cream. Gloria was delighted with the flatness of her abdomen and the way that her abdominal muscles had been tightened as well. I instructed Gloria not to do any abdominal muscle exercises for at least three months in order to prevent ripping the muscle stitches.

Abdominoplasty

After three months, I saw Gloria once again and her results were stunning. She was thrilled and couldn't wait to get into that bikini.

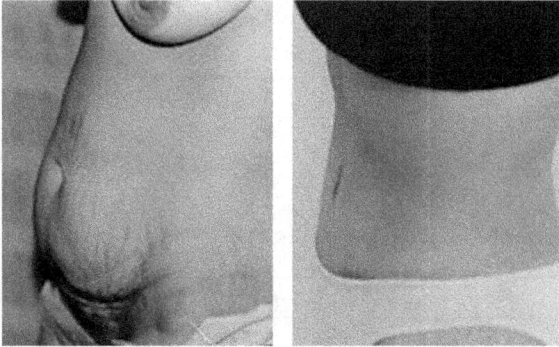

Patient had not only redundant amounts of skin and fat on the lower abdomen, but also had the muscles pulled apart (rectus diastasis). This required tightening of the internal rectus muscle as well as removing the skin and fat to give her an excellent result.

NOTES

_____

_____

_____

_____

_____

_____

_____

_____

_____

_____

_____

_____

_____

_____

_____

_____

_____

_____

_____

_____

_____

_____

_____

_____

_____

_____

_____

_____

_____

_____

_____

_____

NOTES

_____
_____
_____
_____
_____
_____
_____
_____
_____
_____
_____
_____
_____
_____
_____
_____
_____
_____
_____
_____
_____
_____
_____
_____
_____
_____
_____
_____
_____

"IF YOU'RE STRUGGLING TO LOSE WEIGHT, JUST MAKE SURE IT'S NOT BECAUSE THE WORLD WANTS YOU TO."
– MISSY ELLIOTT

CHAPTER 10
Liposuction and Body Contouring

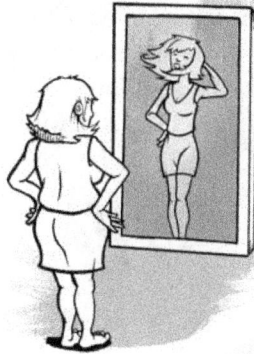

"Our bodies are our gardens to which our wills are gardeners."
– Walt Whitman (1819–1892)

Liposuction is one of the most common cosmetic surgery procedures in the world today. Over the past twenty-five years, physicians have developed the tools and techniques to make liposuction a very safe operation. The results can be spectacular if you are a good candidate for this procedure. However, not everyone is a good candidate.

Liposuction involves the removal of fat cells from localized areas of the body while preserving the nerves, blood vessels, and connective tissue. The location of fat cells within your body determines your overall shape, and this is influenced by heredity. You are born with a certain number of fat cells, and as you gain or lose weight, these cells expand or shrink. The problem is that we don't have much control over where the body deposits these fat cells. Many people find that there are some areas of their body that, no matter how hard they exercise, will always have more fat cells. The only way to correct this problem is through liposuction or the removal of the fat cells.

I will take a moment and caution you. This procedure is not cure-all or a replacement for a good weight-loss program. Diet and exercise are your best defenses against excess fat buildup, and only after you have tried everything you can to lose the additional bulges should a surgical solution be sought.

Liposuction also might not be for you if you have excess skin as well as fat. Merely removing the fat beneath the surface of the skin will not give you a good result. The additional skin will still be left and an alternative path may need to be discussed with your doctor if this is the case.

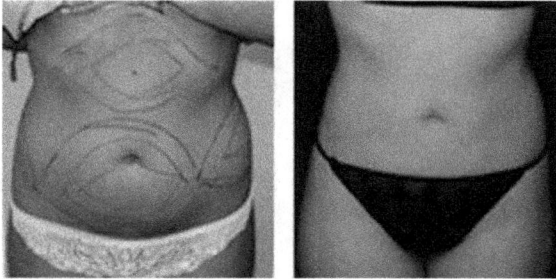

Patient had significant amounts of localized fat deposits, of the upper and lower abdomen and hips. She did extraordinarily well with direct tumescent liposuction technique, removing approximately 1.5 liters of fat.

I frequently get questions from patients who want the lumpy, bumpy appearance of their skin smoothed out. While liposuction can help somewhat, if you have dimpled skin before surgery, the odds are pretty good that you will have dimpled skin afterwards. Remember that this procedure only works with the underlying fat and does not stretch or pull the skin in any way to smooth out wrinkles or bumps. If your goal is to have smoother and less wrinkled skin on certain parts of your body, I would again encourage you to discuss an alternative form of treatment with your doctor. Cellulite is not correctable with any form of liposuction.

I frequently get asked what the difference is between liposculpture and liposuction. The truth of the matter is, they are relatively the same thing. The difference is in the degree of involvement. Again, liposuction involves the removal of fat with a cannula. A cannula is a metal rod with holes at the end that is attached to a vacuum suction in order to suction fat from the deep fat areas of the body. Body contouring is a bit more involved. It entails a combination of procedures, including removal of skin and fat from different parts of the body, such as a tummy tuck, breast lift, and/or breast reduction.

BODY CONTOURING IS A BIT MORE INVOLVED. IT ENTAILS A COMBINATION OF PROCEDURES, INCLUDING REMOVAL OF SKIN AND FAT FROM DIFFERENT PARTS OF THE BODY.

The best candidates for liposuction are women and men who are in excellent overall health, and who have localized fat deposits in specific areas where the skin tension is good. This means that they have fat in the deep fat areas. Under your skin, there are two layers of fat, superficial and deep. We want to liposuction fat mostly from the deep fat areas because it causes less body contour irregularities. Trying to take too much superficial fat may cause dimpling, denting, or disfigurement of the overlying skin.

While the best candidates for liposuction are healthy, it doesn't hurt to be young, either. By young, I mean in your twenties, thirties, or forties, though liposuction can certainly be done at any age if the patient has localized fat deposits in their deep fat, as well as good skin tone. Skin tone plays a major role in determining your final result.

SKIN TONE PLAYS A MAJOR ROLE IN DETERMINING YOUR FINAL RESULT.

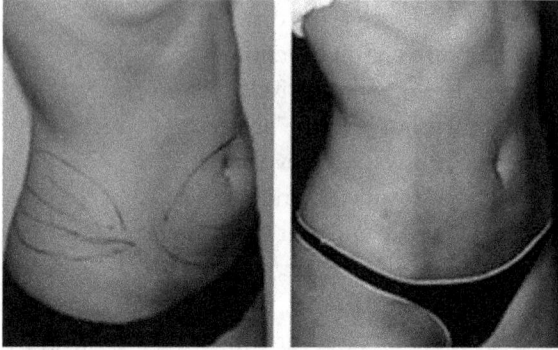

Patient had localized small areas of fat with good skin tone in the lower abdomen and flank areas. These areas were liposuctioned using the tumescent technique with an excellent result.

For example, let's assume our patient is a thirty-year-old woman, has abdominal fat, meaning fat deposits in the lower tummy, hips, and flank areas, and her skin tone is great. She has not had children, but there is a pooch of localized fat that can safely be liposuctioned and the hips can be taken in beautifully, adding a nice curve to the flank area. This can be accomplished without risk of skin laxity or looseness occurring from the liposuctioned areas.

If, on the other hand, the woman is forty, has had three children, and has loose skin around the lower abdominal area, she will probably get a poor result. This is because her main problem is loose skin, not fat. Please remember that skin and fat are completely different issues, and they need to be addressed with different approaches. Loose skin on the abdomen is usually associated with a tummy tuck. Liposuction can only remove a localized fat deposit, such as that small pooch on your stomach that you hate when you look at your body in profile in the mirror. Skin tone is extraordinarily important and is the determining factor for plastic surgeons when they decide whether you will indeed be a good candidate for liposuction.

In terms of the best areas on the body to undergo liposuction, there are several particular regions that take very well to liposuction. I enjoy working on the tummy area, hips, and the flanks as well as the inner and the outer thighs. I feel these are safe zones, and they do very well with liposuctioning. These are normally predictable areas as far as postoperative results.

Be aware that fat is different throughout the various parts of the body. Doctors have found great results with liposuctioning all over the body, including the face. This type of liposuction is often done in combination with face-lift procedures. Liposuction of the lateral breasts can also be performed, with good results in combination with a breast reduction. This reduces some of the fullness and the width on the side of the breast and gives a narrower and less bulging appearance on the side of the chest.

The thighs are also excellent areas for liposuction, especially the saddlebag region. Saddlebags are large pockets of fat on the outside of the thighs that are very noticeable and pronounced. Women really hate this area, and most would love to get rid of it. Interestingly, the fat deposits in the saddlebag area are genetic. Often when the patient comes into my office with this issue, I'll ask her if her mother or sisters have it as well. Normally, the response is yes. This is definitely one of those areas in which diet and exercise are not effective, but this area does do well with liposuction. This is resistant fat that can be suctioned out nicely and smoothed to the point that the woman has a beautiful contour along the lower third of her body.

> THE TUMESCENT TECHNIQUE INFILTRATES FLUID INTO THE AREA TO BE LIPOSUCTIONED

The inner thigh (or the medial thigh) is another area that responds well. But I have to offer a word of caution: this area can be over-suctioned. In this area, the skin can become loose, allowing dents and irregularities to become more exaggerated. A conservative approach is usually best, and I would encourage you to consider liposuction of this area only with a qualified and very experienced board-certified doctor. They must know exactly what they're doing in that particular region, because there is little or no room for error. On the larger parts of the body, such as the hips or lower stomach, some errors may be hardly noticeable, but with the inner thighs, this is not the case.

The most common technique for liposuction is called tumescent liposuction. The tumescent technique infiltrates fluid into the area to be liposuctioned. The fluid that we use for this process has three components.

They are:

1) **Saline solution** – which helps hydrate the fat cells.

2) **Lidocaine** – which has a numbing effect and reduces pain after the operation.

3) **Epinephrine** – which causes the blood vessels to constrict so there is less bleeding.

Using this combination of medication and saline solution makes the liposuction safer because there is less blood loss. There is also much less bruising throughout the areas, leading to a quicker and less painful recovery for the patient.

It is important that your doctor does not suction too much fat at one time. Even with the tumescent technique, there is still blood loss, and the more blood that is lost, the higher the risk. In my practice, we like to limit the amount of aspirate liposuctioned to three to four liters at one time. This is the total volume of fat, blood, and fluid removed. This allows us to make sure that the patient's blood count does not fall below the safe level; if it does, the patient could need a blood transfusion.

Prior to your surgery, your doctor will ask you to have a complete blood count (CBC), which shows your hemoglobin and hematocrit. This is very important because the doctor must determine that you're not anemic prior to surgery, especially if a large liposuction procedure is planned. Again, being anemic could cause you to end up needing a blood transfusion. It is also nice to know your coagulation panel, PT, PTT. This tells the doctor whether or not you're going to clot normally. The ability of a patient to clot well reduces the postoperative bruising and bleeding.

Most of these preoperative blood tests and panels will be performed as part of your surgery. Tests prior to your operation give the entire medical staff a current benchmark of your health. This will ensure a safe operation with a reduced chance of complications. If you are not certain what a particular test is for or why it is needed, just ask your doctor.

ANESTHESIA

For major liposuction cases, I use general anesthesia, and the patient is completely put to sleep. This assures me that the patient will have no memory of the surgery or experience any pain, no matter what part of their body I am working on. It also assures me that the patient will not move on the table, and I can work more carefully without worrying about puncturing a vital structure. For these reasons, I believe that the safest liposuction is always performed under general anesthesia.

> I BELIEVE THAT THE SAFEST LIPOSUCTION IS ALWAYS PERFORMED UNDER GENERAL ANESTHESIA.

After surgery, liposuction patients are placed in compression garments, including abdominal binders and girdles, depending on the areas of the body that were worked on. This allows for a constant and steady compression of these areas, which reduces swelling and bruising. It also smoothes out the tissue and gives a more beautiful, elegant result. Postoperative garments are a must.

Another area of concern that comes up frequently with patients considering liposuction is revisions. It is not uncommon to require a secondary revision after liposuction. Your doctor performs the liposuction procedure mostly by feel. Here again, this is where experience is a must. However, on occasion, there may be a small amount of fat left over in one particular area, which may not be noticeable at first, due to swelling from the initial procedure. If after four to six months these areas have not resolved, they can be taken care of by a small revision surgery to feather them out if necessary.

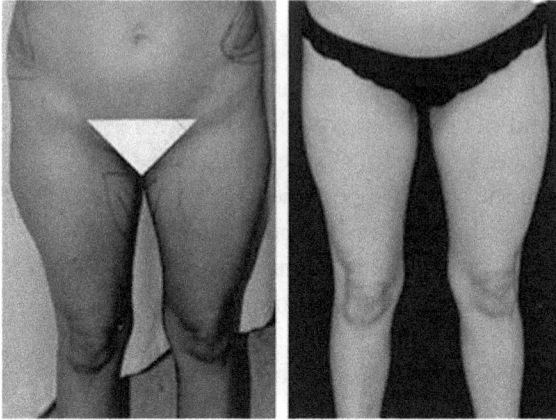

Tumescent liposuction technique performed on the hips and inner and outer thighs. Postoperatively, patient has a nice contour of the thighs, an obvious more sleek appearance with a decrease in the pear-like shape. She also has good skin tone and there is no contour deformities or irregularities.

While liposuction is extremely safe in properly trained hands, you should be aware of what can go wrong. For example, the underlying anatomy of the abdominal area can be in danger. If there is an error, and the cannula enters that area, the patient could develop a perforation or puncture of the intestines, resulting in death. This is one very good reason that a plastic surgeon must be trained in all areas of surgery, not for when things go right, but for when things go wrong. He or she has to be able to diagnose any ensuing complication and know the best course of action.

Liposuction is currently being performed by doctors of every specialty: dermatologists, ER doctors, head and neck doctors, general surgeons, gynecologists, etc. The question you must ask is, are they really properly trained to do this procedure safely? And if there is a complication, will they be able to determine what the problem is and how best to treat it? The answer in most cases is probably no. Even for something as seemingly simple as liposuction, you should choose a qualified, properly trained and experienced board-certified plastic surgeon.

VANESSA'S STORY

I met Vanessa when she was twenty-seven years old. She came to my office extremely self-conscious and unhappy with her body. She felt she had way too much fat in the upper and lower abdominal areas, as well as along her flanks and hips.

Vanessa had very resistant fat along the sides of her thighs, called saddlebags. She wanted liposuction. I talked with Vanessa and examined her carefully. I found that she had good localized deep fat deposit areas that I felt would sculpt out beautifully. Her skin tone was excellent, and she had not yet had any children. We discussed the possibilities that liposuction offered for the various areas and agreed that I would liposuction her hips, flanks, lower and upper abdominal area, and her resistant saddlebags. Vanessa went under general anesthesia, and I sculpted her body using small cannulas with the tumescent liposuction technique.

SHE NO LONGER WORRIES ABOUT THOSE BOTHERSOME SADDLEBAGS OR FEELS SELF-CONSCIOUS ABOUT HER BODY.

One week later, Vanessa's stitches were removed. She remained in a girdle and abdominal binder for six weeks. There was a small amount of residual fat in the belly button area, so I recommended that she undergo some finesse feathering liposuction to revise this area after having healed for three months. I encouraged her to not do this too early in order to prevent possible indentation or contour irregularities.

A few months later, Vanessa underwent the second surgery and, within six weeks, had a beautiful result. She no longer worries about those bothersome saddlebags or feels self-conscious about her body.

LIPOSUCTION WORKSHEET

Before surgery, it is important to understand the technique that will be used for your liposuction procedure. While some patients may be hesitant to discuss things in detail, it is very important to understand exactly what will and won't happen during your surgery.

What technique will be used?

Tumescent technique
Other _____

Will your liposuction procedure be power assisted?

Yes _____ No _____

Check which specific technique the plastic surgeon will be performing.

Specific Technique: _____
Ultrasonic _____
Other _____

How many liters of tumescent fluid/fat aspirate is expected to be removed?

_____

Expect it to be infiltrated. Write this number down. Anything over five liters is considered high volume and may increase risk of complications.

Where will the incisions be made?

Have these marked by the plastic
surgeon in your consultation
prior to your surgery date.

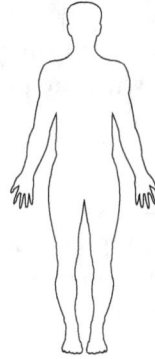

Where will the surgery be performed? Is it in the office, at an ambulatory surgical center, or at the hospital?

_____

Is the facility licensed? _____
Is it Medicare approved? _____
Is it state certified? _____

Does the surgeon use the services of a nurse anesthetist or an anesthesiologist that is a diplomat of the American Board of Anesthesiology? This is very important; there is a difference.

_____

_____

What is the anesthesiologist's name? _____
Number of years in practice? _____
Malpractice record? _____

Have all consent forms been reviewed? Questions should be discussed with the plastic surgeon.

Yes _____ No _____

Examination of the specific areas to be liposuctioned with the plastic surgeon. Twice is preferred, allowing both the patient and surgeon to see any irregularities of the skin, including contour deformities, depressions, and scars from previous surgeries.

Do you have the required postoperative garments?

Abdominal binder, girdles, etc.?
Ask where to buy these or if they will be provided by the plastic surgeon.

Postoperative visits. Write down the dates and times of your postoperative days, including the day of suture removal.

DATE AND TIMES OF FOLLOW-UP APPOINTMENTS

Month	Day	Time
_____	_____	_____
_____	_____	_____
_____	_____	_____
_____	_____	_____
_____	_____	_____

Have you reviewed your postoperative instructions? These should be reviewed with the doctor and consultant. Make sure that all of your questions are thoroughly answered.

NOTES

NOTES

NOTES

_____

_____

_____

_____

_____

_____

_____

_____

_____

_____

_____

_____

_____

_____

_____

_____

_____

_____

_____

_____

_____

_____

_____

_____

_____

_____

_____

_____

_____

_____

_____

_____

"I DON'T THINK OF
ALL THE MISERY, BUT
OF ALL THE BEAUTY
THAT REMAINS."
– ANNE FRANK

CHAPTER 11

Massive Weight Loss

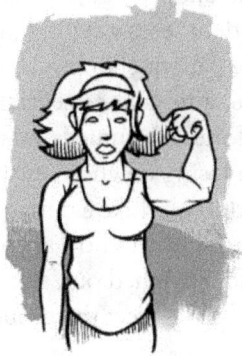

"Great art picks up where nature ends."

– Marc Chagall (1887-1985)

These days, patients are gaining and losing weight more than ever. Some of this weight loss is due to diet and exercise, but more and more patients are finding themselves in the morbidly obese category. This means that they are more than twice their normal body weight. For individuals in this category, there are surgical solutions to help them lose weight. Gastric bypass and gastric banding have become very popular in the last few years, aiding the morbidly obese patient in his or her weight-loss goals. These are not surgeries for the mildly overweight. Most patients who choose these procedures have specific health concerns. The surgery has the potential for life-threatening complications, and the benefits must outweigh the risks to the patient's health.

Gastric bypass procedures, in general, simply make the stomach smaller so there is less room for food, and therefore, patients seem to have less caloric intake. Patients have numerous options for the type of

A PATIENT WHO HAS LOST A MASSIVE AMOUNT OF WEIGHT WILL HAVE SAGGING SKIN ALL OVER THE BODY.

bypass procedure that will suit them, including laparoscopic banding procedures. Some gastric bypass procedures change the size and shape of the stomach, while others restrict absorption of calories by shortening the small intestines. Some do both. There are also banding procedures that allow for adjustment of the stomach as the patient loses weight. No matter what option the patient chooses, all of these surgeries have the same goal, to severely restrict the amount of calories consumed and absorbed into the body.

Once patients begin losing weight, they will notice that while the fat melts away, the skin doesn't. Like a deflated balloon, they are left with large areas of sagging skin and no way to get the skin back into its original position. Once stretched out, the skin will eventually loose its elasticity. The only way to correct the problem is through plastic surgery.

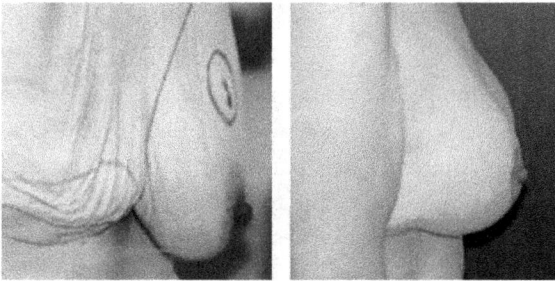

Patient required both increased volume as well as removal of massive amounts of skin. Combination breast augmentation with 500 cc saline implants as well as a formal mastopexy (breast lift) was required to achieve this excellent result.

Here again, this is not to be undertaken lightly. A patient who has lost a massive amount of weight will have sagging skin all over the body. Correcting their problem may involve multiple surgeries and long recuperations. The patient will also have to contend with large scars that are very visible. For many, the trade-off between the removal of massive amount of skin and permanent scars is a worthy exchange. To shed pounds of excess skin is very liberating and allows for greater freedom of movement. For this reason, patients who have endured massive weight loss are often the most satisfied plastic surgery patients.

I usually recommend that a patient undergoing massive weight loss allow their weight to stabilize for at least six months to one year before undergoing plastic surgery. This may seem like a long time, but you have to remember that your body has undergone substantial changes. It is important to maintain a consistent weight and allow your body to adjust to the new you. Often, patients who lose a lot of weight quickly will have trouble finding their ideal weight. If they rush into plastic surgery, then lose or gain more weight, the results could be very disappointing.

Another consideration is maintaining overall health. It is not unusual for weight-loss patients to be deficient in certain vitamins and minerals that are essential for proper healing of wounds. The whole idea of gastric bypass is to get the body to absorb less of what you eat. Unfortunately, this can also mean that you aren't getting some essential nutrients. By taking several months and allowing the body to stabilize, these problems can be monitored and corrected well before surgery.

IT IS VERY IMPORTANT FOR A PATIENT CONSIDERING THESE CHANGES TO HAVE REALISTIC EXPECTATIONS.

The procedures used in massive-weight-loss patients are similar in principle to those surgeries for other patients, what does differ is the extent of the surgery. The surgeon is dealing with large amounts of skin, large areas of the body, and large incisions. The procedures are longer and more strenuous on the patient's body, and the potential for blood loss is greater. The potential for revision is also greater, as the patient will probably need to undergo multiple procedures over time to achieve the best result.

It is very important for a patient considering these changes to have realistic expectations. These are long and complicated procedures that produce amazing changes, but they are not perfect. The surgeon is reconstructing your body and working with what is available. This is one reason it is important to look at before-and-after photos. Your surgeon must have experience with and skill in these reconstructive procedures. You can get a good idea of his expertise by looking closely at the photos and speaking with previous patients who have undergone the same procedure or procedures. You must ask yourself if the results you see on those people would be what you consider good results. Do the people appear symmetrical? Are the scars even and symmetrical or lopsided and placed awkwardly?

Where to have your surgery is a big factor as well. Due to the fact that patients with significant weight loss have more complex surgeries, you must understand that the recovery time will be longer. For this reason, most patients feel more comfortable choosing a surgeon in close proximity to their home. While you may have seen a fantastic surgeon on TV who specializes in the procedures you want, unless you live close to or can plan for an extended stay in the city their practice is, it is impractical to try to commute.

PROCEDURES

After weight loss, loose skin can appear all over the body, under the arms, on the outside of the breasts, and under the armpits, not to mention that the breasts will probably sag significantly. Many patients complain that the skin on their abdominal area becomes very loose, with massive amounts hanging down toward their thighs and interfering with exercise.

They may also experience loose skin around their thighs, both on the inner and outer thighs. Contouring of the inner and outer thighs may require lifting the thighs by removing skin and fat from either the inner and/or outer or both areas. These are procedures that can be associated with massive amounts of scarring, but many patients feel it is a worthy trade-off.

Surgeries that can help with the arms include brachioplasty, which is simply the removal of skin and fat, mostly skin, from the elbow to the upper arm region. This is one area that can look particularly bad if not done well, so be sure the surgeon you are choosing is well trained in this area. Once again, these scars can be quite thick, and some patients may be displeased with them. It is very important that the patient be completely realistic as to their expectations and to the trade-offs associated with a better shape and form.

The massive panniculectomy differs somewhat from an abdominoplasty or tummy tuck. A massive panniculectomy is associated with removal of mass amounts of skin and fat from the abdomen. Liposuction is usually performed on the hip areas at the same time as the panniculectomy is performed, in order to help narrow the sides of the torso and mid-abdominal area.

Before

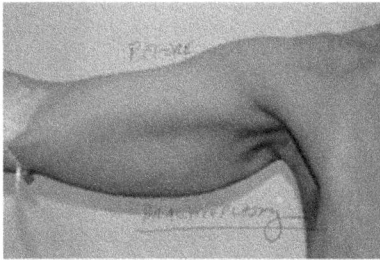 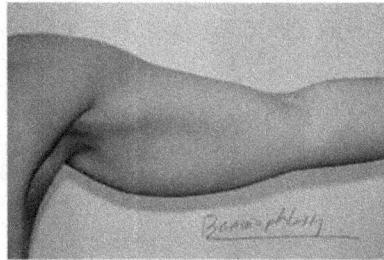

After

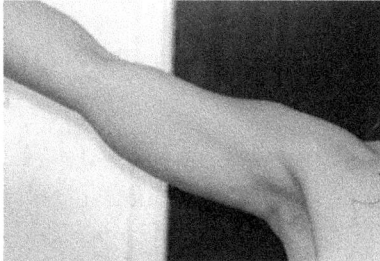 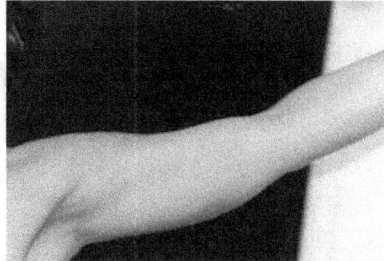

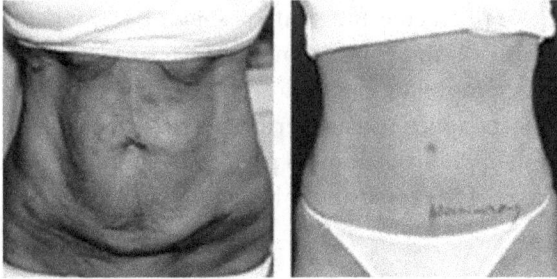

Patient had a significant amount of skin laxity and her muscles had been pulled apart due to pregnancy. She underwent a panniculectomy in order to remove all the redundant skin and has an excellent result. The scar is well hidden beneath the bikini line.

Patients are very happy with these tummy tuck procedures, because not only do they look and feel better in and out of clothing, but they have lost a considerable amount of weight with the removal of skin from their abdominal area. Just like in a breast reduction, in which the reduction of skin and tissue will greatly reduce the heaviness to the chest and back and reduce back pain, neck strain, and grooving along the shoulders, massive panniculectomies aid in the reduction of lower back pain as well as the rashes that these patients often suffer along the suprapubic area, above the pubis.

Liposuction, and body contouring in general, can certainly be performed with other surgical procedures safely. Again, it is vital that the estimated time in the operating room, the amount of time under general anesthesia, and the estimated blood loss from such surgeries all be accounted for prior to considering multiple operations at the same time.

Most importantly, realistic expectations must be maintained by both the doctor and the patient. Remember that in general, when things seem too good to be true, they usually are. If a doctor tells you that you will hardly notice the scars from these operations, they are setting you up for disappointment. The scarring associated with these procedures is always the true trade-off for a better shape, a slimmer size, and a better appearance.

NOTES

_____

_____

_____

_____

_____

_____

_____

_____

_____

_____

_____

_____

_____

_____

_____

_____

_____

_____

_____

_____

_____

_____

_____

_____

_____

_____

_____

_____

_____

_____

_____

NOTES

_____

_____

_____

_____

_____

_____

_____

_____

_____

_____

_____

_____

_____

_____

_____

_____

_____

_____

_____

_____

_____

_____

_____

_____

_____

_____

_____

NOTES

_____
_____
_____
_____
_____
_____
_____
_____
_____
_____
_____
_____
_____
_____
_____
_____
_____
_____
_____
_____
_____
_____
_____
_____
_____
_____
_____
_____
_____
_____

"WE CAN BE
BEAUTIFUL AT ALL
AGES. FEMININE
BEAUTY COMES IN
ALL SHAPES, SIZES,
COLORS, WAYS."
– LAUREN HUTTON

CHAPTER 12
Combination Procedures

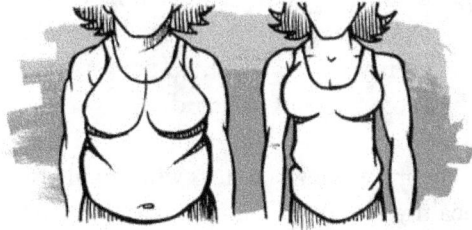

"Beauty lies in the specific looks of a person, rather than the object, because different people feel beauty in different things."

— *Vally*

WHEN YOU SHOULD HAVE THEM, AND WHEN YOU SHOULDN'T.

Whenever you're considering having multiple procedures, several factors need to be taken into consideration. The first factor is the length of surgery time under general anesthesia. The second important consideration is the increased levels of complications or risks with combination procedures. Next, issues regarding the duration of time for your recovery is a very important factor as well.

Statistics from the American Society of Plastic Surgeons in 2004 indicate that thirty-four percent of patients undergoing plastic surgery have combination or multiple procedures performed. Procedures can be combined in many different ways. In terms of body sculpting, breast augmentation can be performed with breast lift if the blood supply is excellent and can be maintained. Breast augmentation can also be performed with liposuction of different body parts as long

SAFETY IS
THE MOST
IMPORTANT
CONSIDERATION
OF ANY PLASTIC
SURGERY
PROCEDURE.

as the amount of liposuction aspirate is kept to a reasonable amount. Breast augmentation can also be performed in conjunction with an abdominoplasty or tummy- tuck procedure as long as the estimated blood loss, and the duration of time under general anesthesia is reasonable (less than five or six hours is usually considered standard).

Facial-plasty procedures can also be performed with multiple ancillary injectable procedures as well as with small body sculpting procedures in healthy patients. The main reason to combine surgical procedures is to allow for a better final result, to have only one anesthesia performed, and for cost containment, as a patient should incur only one fee for the operating room and the anesthesiologist.

Safety is the most important consideration of any plastic surgery procedure. At no time should a patient's safety be at risk while undergoing multiple operations. As with any plastic surgery procedure, it is important that the following factors be confirmed prior to surgery. With multiple procedures and the increased risks they entail, it is absolutely vital to ascertain the following:

1. That your doctor is trained and board certified with the American Board of Plastic Surgery.

2. That the ambulatory surgery center is certified with either AAAASF, Medicare licensed, and/or state licensed.

3. That the anesthesiologist is board certified with the American Board of Anesthesiology.

4. That the patient has had a very thorough history and physical, including laboratories. All systemic or medical illnesses should be cleared prior to surgery by a specialist as necessary.

5. The plastic surgeon should take a detailed history and physical examination of the patient. Family history should also be obtained, including history of diabetes, high blood pressure, auto-immune diseases, as well as medications that the patient is taking, including oral contraceptives, hormone replacement therapy, and herbal supplements, which can increase your risk for complications.

Other risk factors can include:

1. Morbid obesity or being overweight.
2. History of cancer, infections.
3. History of deep veinous thrombosis, history of clotting such as pulmonary embolus, or bleeding disorders such as von Willebrand's disease.

Patients with these risk factors should always undergo thorough testing by hematology. Once cleared, they should still have pneumatic compressive garments intraoperatively and possibly wear elastic stockings after the operation.

Interesting statistics from a 1997 survey by the American Society of Plastic Surgeons indicate that the rate of serious complications is less than one-half of one percent when reviewing 400,000 operations performed in outpatient accredited facilities. The mortality rate was 1 in 57,000. This includes patients who had multiple procedures. So with the right precautions, multiple procedures can be performed safely.

In discussing liposuction, the methods and the amount of fat removed for liposuction has always been controversial. Large-volume liposuction is indicated when over 5,000 cc of aspirate of both fat and fluid are removed. Amounts of fat and fluid that exceed this ceiling can increase risk of electrolyte imbalances, cardiac arrhythmias, and other post-operative medical complications. The local anesthesia and the fluid, normal saline or lactated Ringer's solution, can cause electrolyte disturbances when given using the tumescent technique in very large volumes. As a result, these patients must undergo very strict anesthesia monitoring for fluid status, as well as for blood loss and aspirate amounts. They must also have extended postoperative monitoring with large-volume liposuction techniques as a precaution.

BODY SCULPTING AND COMBINATION PROCEDURES

Once the patient has been cleared, it is then absolutely essential to review the anatomy and the details of the operation, including the anticipated estimated blood loss; and the duration of time under general anesthesia in determining safety for the patient.

With respect to general anesthesia, there has been much controversy as to the increased risk associated with remaining under general anesthesia for more than five or six hours. Patients who will require surgical time over this period should certainly have clearance from specialists, as well as EKGs, blood tests, etc.

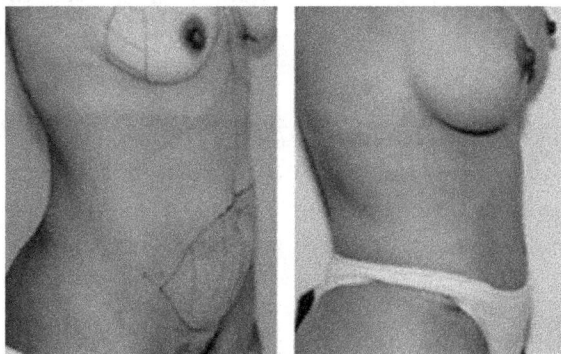

Patient had 375 cc saline implants placed behind the muscle and a full abdominoplasty for an excellent body makeover.

Breast augmentations are often performed with mastopexies of different types, including nipple lifts, vertical lifts, and formal mastopexies, at the same time. The blood supply is absolutely essential when performing a breast lift at the same time as an augmentation. The board-certified plastic surgeon has the experience to determine the safety issues associated with these procedures, realizing that when a breast augmentation and a lift is done at the same time the risk of scarring increases. Therefore, it may be better in certain circumstances to stage the operations, doing the breast augmentation first and the mastopexy several months later, once the tension is reduced.

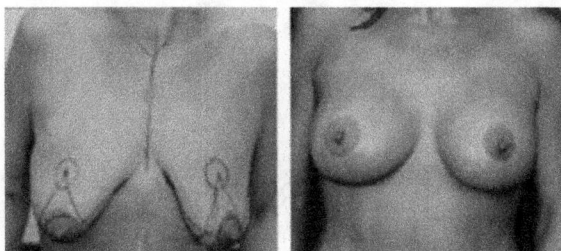

Patient underwent a formal mastopexy (breast lift) with implants in order to regain fullness. The implants are 465 cc high profile saline and a total breast lift was performed to remove skin and bring the nipple areolar complexes back to their normal positions.

Breast augmentations can also be performed with liposuctions. These liposuctions may be done on the abdomen, thighs, and other areas. The amount of fat removed should be reduced when doing combination procedures in order to reduce total estimated blood loss and duration of time under general anesthesia. Breast augmentations and tummy tucks can also be performed together in healthy patients. Tummy tucks are most often performed with liposuction, especially at the iliac crest roll or hip areas, in order to reduce and narrow the lower abdominal area and give a more streamlined appearance.

In terms of facial procedures, depending upon the amount of time of the facial procedure in certain circumstances, face-lifts, brow lifts, and eyelid surgeries can be performed concurrently with breast augmentations, tummy tucks, or liposuction procedures.

There are many commonly performed noninvasive procedures that include injections of fillers, including Restylane, collagen, Radiesse, as well as injections of Botox into facial muscles. These can be performed with body sculpting procedures. Care should be taken when performing facial operations and laser treatments on tissue or skin that has already been dissected or stretched due to the increased risk of burning, skin necrosis, and blood-supply problems. A board—certified plastic surgeon will have the knowledge to keep you out of trouble with these specific procedures.

"THE WORD "**SCAR**"
WAS DERIVED FROM
THE GREEK WORD
ESCHARA, MEANING
FIREPLACE."

CHAPTER 13
The Truth about Scars

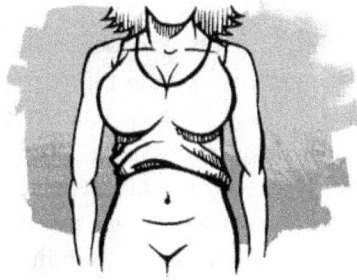

"There is something beautiful about all scars of whatever nature. A scar means the hurt is over, the wound is closed and healed, done with."

– Harry Crew

Scars are areas of fibrous tissue that replace normal skin (or other tissue) after destruction of some of the dermis. A scar results from the biologic process of wound repair in the skin and other tissues of the body. Thus, scarring is a natural part of the healing process. With the exception of very minor lesions, every wound (e.g. after accident, disease, or surgery) results in some degree of scarring.

Scar tissue is not identical to the tissue which it replaces and is usually of inferior functional quality. For example, scars in the skin are less resistant to ultraviolet radiation, and sweat glands and hair follicles do not grow back within scar tissue.

A scar is a natural part of the healing process. Skin scars occur when the deep, thick layer of skin (the dermis) is damaged. The worse the damage is, the worse the scar will be.

Most skin scars are flat, pale and leave a trace of the original injury which caused them. The redness that often follows an injury to the skin is not a scar, and is generally not permanent. The time it takes for it to go away may, however, range from a few days to, in some serious and rare cases, several years. Various treatments can speed up the process.

Scars form differently based on the location of the injury on the body and the age of the person who was injured.

To mend the damage, the body has to lay down new collagen fibres (a naturally occurring protein which is produced by the body).

This process results in a fortuna scar. Because the body cannot re-build the tissue exactly as it was, the new scar tissue will have a different texture and quality than the surrounding normal tissue. An injury does not become a scar until the wound has completely healed.

Two types of scars are the result of the body overproducing collagen, which causes the scar to be raised above the surrounding skin. **Hypertrophic scars** take the form of a red raised lump on the skin, but do not grow beyond the boundaries of the original wound, and they often improve in appearance after a few years. **Keloid scars** are a more serious form of scarring, because they can carry on growing indefinitely into a large, tumorous (although benign) growth.

Both hypertrophic and keloid scars are more common on younger and darker skinned people. They can occur on anyone, but some people have a genetic susceptibility to these types of scarring. They can be caused by surgery or an accident.

Although they can be a cosmetic problem, keloid scars are only inert masses of collagen and therefore completely harmless, painless, and non-contagious. They tend to be most common on the shoulders and chest. Keloid scars are most common among people of Asian or African descent.

Alternately, a scar can take the form of a sunken recess in the skin, which has a pitted appearance. These are caused when underlying structures supporting the skin, such as fat or muscle, are lost.

Scars can also take the form of stretched skin. These are caused when the skin is stretched rapidly, for instance during pregnancy, adolescent growth spurts, the placement of implants, massive weight loss, or when skin is put under tension during the healing process. This type of scar usually improves in appearance after a few years.

TREATMENTS FOR SKIN SCARS

No scar can ever be completely removed. They will always leave a trace, but their appearance can be improved by a number of means, including:.

Creams containing Vitamin E, as well as dietary sources such as wheat germ, nuts, vegetable oils, eggs and green vegetables, can help speed up the healing process, and lessen the appearance of any scar afterwards. Cocoa butter cream can be used to help heal scars, and to prevent the formation of keloid scars.

Studies show that regular use of copper peptides can help remove abnormal skin cells along with exfoliation, alpha hydroxy acids, and beta hydroxy acids over the course of a year. Scar tissue is abnormal collagen, and the skin produces it as a quick fix for the skin to prevent infection. It takes the stem cells in the skin time to grow normal collagen.

Surgical Approach

Any surgical scar removal will always leave a new scar that will take up to two years to mature. Surgery can never remove a scar but can be used to alter its alignment or shape to make it less noticeable.

In the case of hypertrophic or keloid scarring, surgery is not recommended, as there is a high risk of re-occurrence of possibly worse scarring following surgery.

Laser Surgery & Resurfacing

The redness of scars may be reduced by treatment with a vascular laser. It has been theorised that removing layers of skin with a carbon dioxide laser may help flatten scars, although this treatment is still experimental.

The Fraxel laser was recently FDA approved for the treatment of acne scars.

Steroid injections

A long term course of steroid injections under medical supervision, into the scar may help flatten and soften the appearance of keloid or hypertrophic scars.

The steroid is injected into the scar itself; since very little is absorbed into the blood stream, side effects of this treatment are minor. This treatment is repeated at 4-6 week intervals.

Pressure garments

Pressure garments should be used only under supervision by a medical professional. They are most often used for burn scars that cover a large area, this treatment is only effective on recent scars.

Radiotherapy

Low-dose, superficial radiotherapy, is used to prevent re-occurrence of severe keloid and hypertrophic scarring. It is usually effective, but only used in extreme cases due to the risk of long-term side effects.

Dermabrasion

Dermabrasion involves the removal of the surface of the skin with specialist equipment and usually involves a general anaesthetic. It is useful with raised scars, but is less effective when the scar sunken below the surrounding skin.

Collagen injections

Collagen injections can be used to raise sunken scars to the level of surrounding skin. Its effects are however temporary, and it needs to be regularly repeated. There is also a risk in some people of an allergic reaction.

Other treatments

There are also a number of *gel sheets* available which are usually made from silicone, which can help to flatten and soften raised scars if worn regularly. Silicone, pressure, occlusion, topical cortisone and vitamin E have all been shown to decrease the collagen that forms scars. Patches and pads help but are unsightly so people tend to quit. A popular treatment among plastic surgeons is Scarfade, a silicone gel that improves the appearance of scars and prevents abnormal or excessive scar formation. Also chemical peels performed by a dermatologist using glycolic acid can be used to minimize acne scarring.

NOTES

NOTES

_____

_____

_____

_____

_____

_____

_____

_____

_____

_____

_____

_____

_____

_____

_____

_____

_____

_____

_____

_____

_____

_____

_____

_____

_____

_____

_____

_____

_____

"SHE GOT HER LOOKS
FROM HER FATHER.
HE'S A PLASTIC
SURGEON."
– GROUCHO MARX

CHAPTER 14
The Truth about Plastic Surgery

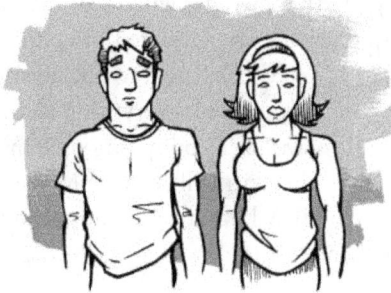

"Beauty is a sign of intelligence."

– Andy Warhol

1. BREAST AUGMENTATION SURGERY

In general, most women are very happy with the results of their enhancement surgery. However, with time (usually many years), changes will happen with the breasts. Gravity will always continue to take its toll upon the entire body, especially the breasts. Wearing an under-wire bra during the day and a sports bra during the evenings may help to reduce the continued descent and recurrent sagginess of the breasts. However, this cannot guarantee that over time a woman's breasts will not sag again.

I've seen in my practice that as women age, they may have more sagginess to the breasts. In fact, bottoming out of the implant or a case in which the implant ends up low and the nipple ends up high on top of the breast can even occur, especially when women do not

A BIG DETERMINING FACTOR IN HOW WELL A WOMAN'S BREAST IMPLANTS LOOK OVER TIME IS HER WILLINGNESS TO WEAR SUPPORTIVE CLOTHING AND BRAS

wear supportive bras. The weight of the breast implants themselves, especially the larger implants, may cause the muscle and fatty tissue to give out and cease to keep the implant in the proper location. In other words, when a woman commits to having a breast augmentation surgery, she must understand that changes will occur over time and often those changes are not complementary.

What I wish to emphasize is that as we all get older, everything changes in life, and a woman's body is not exempt just because she had plastic surgery. The skin will become looser, the tissue may atrophy, glandular tissue may be reduced, and more fatty tissue may develop, causing the implant to droop.

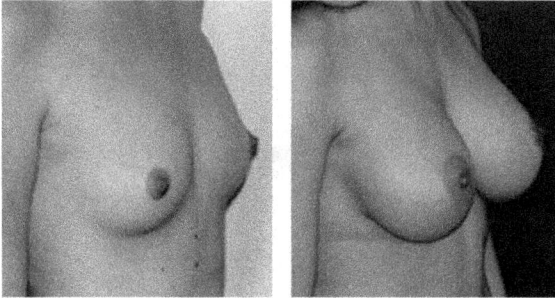

Patient started out with 34A breasts and decided to become a full C, 440 cc high profile, smooth round saline implants were placed behind the muscle using the dual plane technique. The periareolar approach was used giving the patient a natural looking result.

The time that this takes to occur is not standardized, therefore, one woman could develop sagginess to her breasts as soon as one year after surgery, while another woman may still look great ten years later. A lot of it has to do with the genetic content of a woman's breasts and the structure of the tissue itself. It is also dependent on the skin and how well it holds up over time. A big determining factor in how well a woman's breast implants look over time is her willingness to wear supportive clothing and bras, which will help to maintain the implant in an elevated position.

Scar tissue is also something of which women need to be very aware. Unpredictable scar tissue is quite common. I see it often in my practice, due to the fact that we specialize in breast surgery and breast revision surgery. Scar tissue can occur from surgery with any plastic surgeon. There is absolutely no guarantee that **any** plastic surgeon can operate so that a woman will not develop scar tissue. New and different medications that are not yet FDA approved, but which are starting to be used, may help to reduce scar tissue formation. However, we do not know what the side effects of these medications are in terms of toxicity, and therefore, until the FDA has approved those products, you may want to use currently approved methods.

Scar tissue can occur at any time after the augmentation has been performed, not just the first few months. As soon as the capsule forms around the implant, which occurs within weeks, trauma to the capsule can reinitiate the process of hardening and scar tissue formation. Sometimes, if found early, massage and vitamins may reduce or prevent progressive hardening; however, once it becomes painful and the breast implant becomes distorted by constriction of the hardened capsule around the bag, it usually will require a secondary surgery.

But, you must understand that removing the scar tissue or releasing it cannot guarantee that the scar tissue will not reform in the future. I want to make it clear that once you commit to having breast augmentation surgery, it is quite likely that you will end up having to have another surgery sometime down the road for one reason or another.

WE LIVE ON A GRAVITATIONAL PLANET; EVERYTHING SAGS.

It is important to remember before you consider having the breast enhancement operation that there are real long-term issues that must be dealt with, and while we do have solutions for those issues, you must be ready and willing to undergo maintenance of your enhanced breasts in the future. Understanding this will help you to have a positive outlook toward this operation and realistic expectations.

Another problem relates to recurrent sagginess, the laxity of the skin. With time, the breasts will sag again; it is inevitable. We live on a gravitational planet; everything sags. Wearing supportive bras will certainly help to keep your lifted breasts in place, but that is no guarantee that they will remain there. Your genes determine the quality of your skin and the amount of fat or glandular tissue in your breasts. If you have a lot of stretch marks on your breasts, and your skin does not have a lot of good tensile strength, there is a pretty good chance that your breasts are going to sag with time. Once again, be realistic with your expectations.

Also, understand that somewhere down the road you certainly may require a revision breast lift, with more skin removed, the areolar lifted again and the breast tightened. One does not know when that may occur. Some women's breasts become quite saggy or have increased recurrent laxity in a relatively short period of time. Others may not have a problem for twenty or thirty years. It depends on your genes.

> NO PLASTIC SURGEON CAN GUARANTEE THE FINAL APPEARANCE OF A SCAR.

2. BREAST LIFT MASTOPEXY

A breast lift operation is an excellent surgery in that it elevates, enhances, and lifts the breasts while helping to boost the woman's self-esteem. Unfortunately, breast lifts and breast reduction patients must trade the positive effects of these surgeries for the scars that they inevitably leave. Whether a lollypop scar or true anchor scar, many scars can heal in an unpredictable manner. No plastic surgeon can guarantee the final appearance of a scar. The truth of all truths is that scarring is unpredictable within nature, and no final outcome is certain. Granted, the technical ability of the plastic surgeon is extremely important. However, even the most beautifully sutured incision can heal with terrible results, no matter how much effort is put into that closure.

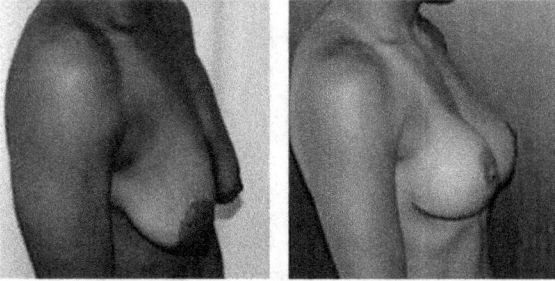

Patient underwent a formal mastopexy (breast lift) with 425 cc high profile saline implants placed under the muscle, using the dual plane technique. Patient also required an areolar reduction.

Please remind yourself to be realistic. Look at hundreds of pictures of scars, as well as actual patients from the surgeon's office, if possible, to prepare yourself, and make sure that you are truly ready to trade those scars for better-shaped and lifted breasts.

3. COMBINATION OF BREAST AUGMENTATION WITH BREAST LIFTS

This combination of operations seems to lead to the highest incidence of recurrent sagginess. When you're having a large implant placed under the muscle and lifting the breasts at the same time, that heavy implant will eventually cause the skin to droop once again. I have seen this in my practice on numerous occasions in patients who've had augmentation lifts done by excellent surgeons. A woman who decides to have a breast enhancement and a lift at the same time needs to understand that even though the breasts look beautiful three months after surgery, or even a few years later, her breasts may be saggy again, and she may require a revision breast lift.

THE SIZE OF THE IMPLANT YOU HAVE PLACED IS A MAJOR INDICATOR OF HOW QUICKLY YOUR BREASTS MAY SAG AFTER SURGERY.

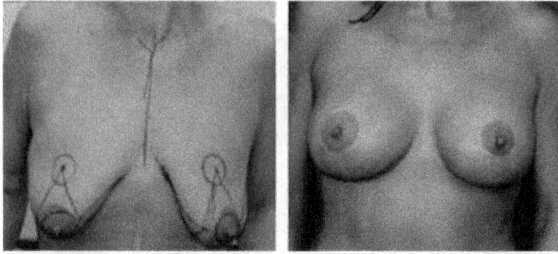

Patient underwent combination breast augmentation and breast lift surgery. Patient previously had undergone a gastric bypass procedure with massive weight loss of over 100 pounds. In order to achieve the desired results patient required increased volume. Saline implants were placed in the dual plane behind the muscle as well as a formal mastopexy (breast lift) performed with repositioning of the nipple and removal of redundant skin.

The size of the implant you have placed is a major indicator of how quickly your breasts may sag after surgery. The larger the implant, the sooner you're going to need to have a lift once again. You may want to consider going with a smaller implant with your breast lift, in order to lengthen the time between surgeries in the future.

4. BREAST REDUCTION

The truth about breast reduction is that it is one of the most life changing operations that patients can have. These patients are also some of the most grateful patients that I see in my practice. Functional pain, neck strain, shoulder grooving, back pain, and rashes are greatly relieved or completely eliminated altogether by breast reduction surgery. Remember, though, that breast reductions, especially very large reductions, can require multiple staged surgeries. The truth of the matter is that often after the first surgery, the breasts may look somewhat flat or boxy in appearance. The sides of the breasts often need to be trimmed at a secondary stage or even liposuctioned. This is very frequently done in a second surgery. As a result, all of our patients are informed up front that multiple stage surgeries are often required on breast reductions, both in order to allow for a normal shape of the breast and to reduce the flattening and boxy appearance of the side of the chest.

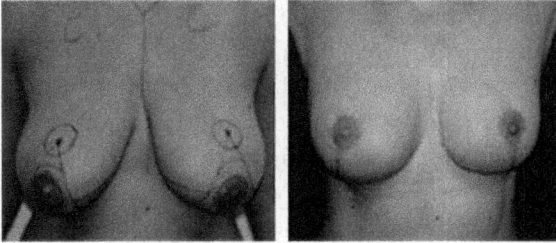

Patient underwent a moderate size breast reduction, approximately 350 grams of tissue were removed per breast, the Wise-pattern technique was performed. Notice, the nipple positioning is centralized within her breast.

Scarring on breast reductions can be significant. While they may look very nice for the first few weeks and/or months, they may change. Scars spread over time, and once again no plastic surgeon can guarantee that your scar is going to look perfect at any time. Early on, you may develop keloid or hypertrophic scarring (thickening of the scars), which can become painful due to nerve growth into the scars. You may want to consider a consultation with a dermatologist who can inject steroids such as Kenalog into the scars helping to flatten elevated scarring.

Be wary of the amount of breast tissue removed during your breast reduction. Make sure you and your plastic surgeon are one-hundred percent in agreement as to the final size of your breasts. It is very easy for your breasts to come out too small or to be reduced to a level with which you are unhappy. Simply looking at pictures alone may not be adequate for your plastic surgeon to understand what size you want. In my practice, I always believe it is important to err on

> MAKE SURE YOU AND YOUR PLASTIC SURGEON ARE ONE-HUNDRED PERCENT IN AGREEMENT AS TO THE FINAL SIZE OF YOUR BREASTS.

the side of taking less tissue rather than too much in order to allow a woman to maintain her feminine appearance, but this is a decision that the patient and the doctor should discuss during multiple consultations regarding a breast reduction.

Interestingly, patients will come into my office, evaluate their breasts, and find that they really are not a candidate for breast reduction, but rather a breast lift with a very small reduction of tissue removed mostly from the outer portions of the breasts in order to reduce the lateral fullness. In fact, breast lifts alone often will give the appearance of a reduced size breast with over a cup size reduction. Simply removing skin alone in many patients will not only lift the breast, but also give it a slightly smaller appearance. Saggy, atrophied, fatty breast tissue with a lot of loose skin can appear quite large in size, but sometimes is really not, and when the breast is lifted and the skin is removed, the breast is much smaller than what was anticipated. It is exceedingly important that you and your plastic surgeon be very careful in your consideration of the amount of tissue you decide to remove to attain your final size.

It is imperative to have a mammogram prior to a breast reduction procedure. You may also want to consider an ultrasound as well. Once tissue is removed and the remaining tissue is rearranged, it is important to have a preoperative baseline map of what your breasts looked like prior to the operation, especially if there are any types of masses, calcifications, or lesions that the radiologists might want to review at a later date. Board—certified plastic surgeons will send all tissue taken from the breasts to pathology to ensure that there is no evidence of cancer within any of the specimens. It is also a good idea to get a copy of your pathology report after surgery for your own records.

5. ABDOMINOPLASTY

In general, it is very important that you have realistic expectations. Some women come to my office to have a tummy tuck only to find they have what is called intra-abdominal fat or a protuberant abdomen. These women do not always have the best results from an abdominoplasty. Even though they have a lot of extra skin below the belly button or umbilicus, they still appear to have a bulge after the surgery. It is important that if you hear the word "intra-abdominal fat" that you understand that you will never have a flat stomach.

It is absolutely not going to happen, even with tightening of the abdominal muscles internally. This fat is entangled within your abdominal cavity, so merely tightening the muscles over it won't eliminate your bulge. I am only addressing tissue outside the muscle with a tummy tuck; I am not addressing anything within the abdominal cavity. That is an area not to be touched during any elective operation at any time.

> IT IS EXTREMELY IMPORTANT THAT YOU UNDERSTAND THAT MULTIPLE SURGERIES MAY BE REQUIRED TO GET YOUR FINAL, DESIRED RESULT

Scarring from abdominoplasties can range from excellent to horrible. As I have stated many times, there is no guarantee as to the final appearance of your scar. If you do develop a keloid and/or hypertrophic scarring, once again I recommend a dermatologist inject steroids early on if you are a candidate. Speak with a well-informed board-certified dermatologist who does injections of Kenalog or other steroids.

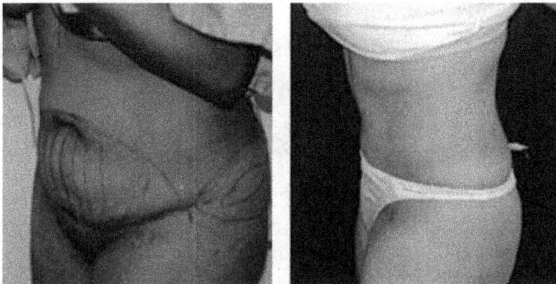

Patient underwent both an abdominoplasty as well as liposuctioning of the iliac crest rolls or hips to allow her a beautiful flattened stomach as well as narrowing of her hips.

Abdominoplasty surgeries, especially large ones, often require staged operations such as we described in breast reductions. Sometimes we must perform liposuction of the upper abdominal wall and the flanks. I prefer not to do these during the original surgery because of the risk of blood-supply problems to the lower flaps, which could cause death of the skin. It is extremely important that you understand that multiple surgeries may be required to get your final, desired result and in order to have a safe and predictable outcome. Discuss this in detail with your plastic surgeon. In general, women who are really quite thin, who have a lot of loose skin, and who don't have a lot of extra fat can usually undergo one operation with an excellent result. On the other hand, women who have increased fat or lipodystrophy of the upper abdominal area, flanks, and hips often require a full abdominoplasty. Several months later after the wounds are completely healed, liposuction of the entire abdominal area, upper and lower abdomen, hips, flanks, etc., is necessary to allow a reduction of the flap and thinning out of the abdominal wall and hips and flanks. This creates a beautiful, more tapered look.

6. LIPOSUCTION

Liposuction is one of the most commonly performed surgeries. It is exceedingly important that you are the right candidate for liposuction. If you have a lot of loose skin, you're probably not a good candidate. If the doctor is still attempting liposuction, you probably should seek another opinion. Liposuction should be done under general anesthesia. I believe it is the safest approach possible, because the patient is completely under and is not going to be able to move during the operation. Therefore, the plastic surgeon can suction in the safe planes without ending up in the wrong place. Liposuctioning too deeply or aggressively can result in perforations of the intestines or other organs. Liposuctioning too close to the skin can leave you with track marks, dents, and contour deformities, which may be absolutely impossible to repair.

LIPOSUCTIONING TOO CLOSE TO THE SKIN CAN LEAVE YOU WITH TRACK MARKS, DENTS, AND CONTOUR DEFORMITIES

Another important point to consider about liposuction is revision, which is also very common. It may be required. If you have realistic expectations as to the final result, you should be happy. Patients frequently ask, "How many pounds are you going to remove?" Surgeons don't measure in pounds for liposuction, it is not an operation for removing pounds of fat. Liposuction should be done to sculpt the body. Once a woman is at a baseline weight, it is the best time to try to remove resistant fat deposits in the various areas of the abdomin, the thighs , and the lateral breast areas. These are areas that do well, and they are the safest areas for predictable results. Remember that liposuction is never a substitution for weight loss.

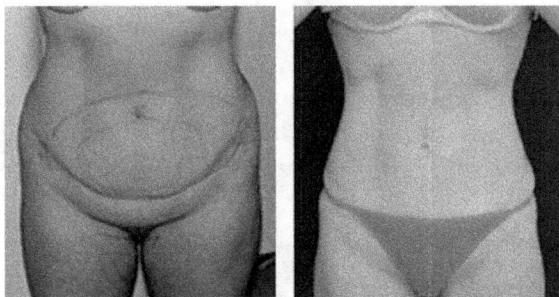

Patient underwent liposuctioning of her lower abdomen. Although she has a mild to moderate amount of loose skin on the lower abdomen, she was not a candidate for an abdominoplasty as the patient was hoping to have children in the near future. Therefore, she desired to have straight liposuction at the time, 1.25 liters was removed from her lower abdomen and inner and outer thigh areas.

Patients should try to reduce their problem areas with diet and exercise prior to considering liposuction. It is also important to understand that after the surgery, small areas called fibrotic fat areas, which are associated with little islands of fat left over from tracking in different directions and different planes with the cannula, may lead to hardened fibrotic lumps. This is usually resolved with time. Massaging with vitamin E, cocoa butter, and other such products is useful and ultrasonic manipulation may be advised as well if the area is quite hard. These areas almost always resolve on their own, but once they have resolved, every six months you should revisit your plastic surgeon and evaluate the entire area that was sculpted, looking for any divots, dents, irregularities, or contour deformities that may appear. These can easily be corrected with very small cannulas and/or fat grafting if necessary.

It is important that your doctor not be so aggressive that he leaves you with indentations. You must find a plastic surgeon who is well trained and experienced in liposuction and who performs liposuction several times a week. There truly is an art form to doing this procedure! It is not simply hacking with a cannula and sucking fat out, but rather knowing exactly where the planes to suction the fat are and how much fat to suction. It is truly an artistic challenge, and it requires a great deal of skill by the doctor.

Pressure garments are an absolute must in my practice. You should expect to wear these garment for at least six to eight weeks minimum to allow the tissue and swelling to resolve. This assists with creating an even contour of the areas that were sculpted.

WORKSHEETS AND NOTES

This section will give you the worksheets from various chapters in this book and also a place to write your notes and questions as you begin your journey into plastic surgery.

SCREENING WORKSHEET

After you've done your research, you will want to prepare yourself as best as you can for your appointments. It is absolutely vital that you take a worksheet of all the important questions with you, so that you and the doctor can go through it point by point and not leave anything out. This will be the most valuable tool that you will have to assist you in making an informed, educated decision.

• Name of doctor.

  _____

• Specialty?

  _____

• Is the doctor a diplomat of the American Board of Plastic Surgery?

  yes _____   no _____

  If not, why? _____

• Number of procedures performed per year of the specific procedure that you are looking to have done. For example, if you're having breast augmentation, how many augmentations has the doctor performed
  per week?   _____
  per month? _____
  per year?   _____

- Number of years in practice? _____

- Malpractice lawsuits? Number of lawsuits _____,
  and outcomes. _____

- Surgical approach used for the procedure that you are considering.
  (This is very important; there are various techniques that can be
  used for each procedure. For example, for breast augmentation
  there are different kinds of incisions: peri-areolar, through the
  belly button, under the armpit, over the muscle, under the muscle,
  etc. You need to know which technique is the safest and which will
  provide you with the best possible results.)

  _____
  _____
  _____

- Photographs. Review as many before-and-after photos as possible.
  Be sure to look at the height, weight, and body dimensions of each
  patient and what the results look like after. Do they look "done,"
  or are they natural looking? Does the doctor have the ability to
  make you look the way you want to look?

  _____
  _____
  _____

- Anesthesia. Does the surgeon use the services of a nurse
  anesthetist or an anesthesiologist that is a diplomat of the
  American Board of Anesthesiology? This is very important; there
  is a difference.

  _____
  _____

  What is the anesthesiologist's name? _____
  Number of years in practice? _____
  Malpractice record? _____

- Where will the surgery be performed? Is it in the office, at an ambulatory surgical center, or at the hospital?

  _____

  Is the facility licensed?   _____
  Is it Medicare approved?   _____
  Is it state certified?   _____

- Will the procedure be done on an outpatient or inpatient basis?

  _____

  If done at an outpatient facility, what is the reciprocity agreement with nearby hospitals for emergency purposes?

  _____

  Name of Hospital: _____

  Is there a contract with paramedics and ambulance services for emergencies?

  _____

- Revisions. What will your responsibility be for revisions?

  _____

  Will you be responsible for operating room fees? _____
  Anesthesia fees? _____
  Or for a total fee once again? _____

- What is your financial responsibility if something goes wrong after your initial surgery? _____

  If you develop an infection, have a deflation of an implant, or develop hypertrophic scarring? _____

- Nursing staff and surgical scrub technicians. All of these people will be a part of your surgery. Are they certified and/or licensed?

  _____

  ICU certified? _____
  How many years have they been with the doctor and at the facility?

  _____

- Postoperative care. What will the follow-up appointments be like?

  _____

  How many follow-up visits will you need to make during your recovery process? _____

  When will your stitches (sutures) be removed? _____
  By whom? _____

- Physician coverage and after-hours contact. How will you reach the surgeon after-hours if you have an issue?

  _____

  _____

  If your doctor is not available, how is coverage for him/her handled? _____

- What should you expect during the recovery process?

  _____

  _____

  _____

  Will you receive a list of do's and don'ts to have on hand while you're recovering?

  _____

NOTES

_____

_____

_____

_____

_____

_____

_____

_____

_____

_____

_____

_____

_____

_____

_____

_____

_____

_____

_____

_____

_____

_____

_____

_____

_____

_____

_____

_____

_____

_____

BREAST AUGMENTATION SURGERY WORKSHEET

Prior to your surgery there are a number of items that you **must** discuss with your doctor. I have provided the following worksheet to help guide you through this process. You should bring a copy with you to each consultation.

APPROACH OF PROCEDURE

Where will the incisions be made?

Periareolar
Trans-Umbilical
Trans-axillary
Other _____

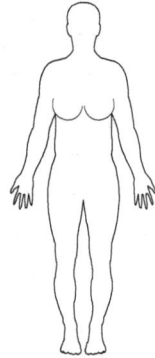

Where will the implant be placed?

Behind the Muscle
Above the Muscle

What kind of implant will be used?

Saline
Silicone
Other _____

What size of implant will be used?

_____ cc
Filled to? _____ cc
Manufacturer? Inamed, Mentor or other _____

Will a concurrent breast lift be performed?

_____

If so, what type? _____
Periareolar, vertical, or anchor scar

What are the credentials of the anesthesiologist?

Are they board certified? Yes or No

What is the accreditation of the ambulatory surgical center?

_____

Be sure to carefully review all consent forms and documentation.

Additional Questions

_____

_____

NOTES

POST-OPERATIVE WORKSHEET

Be sure to keep your post-operative instructions and paperwork for future reference. This can be very instrumental in the event you require revision surgery at a later date. This information will allow your doctor to understand your prior surgery so that you may receive optimal treatment.

Items you keep on file:

Implant manufacturer _____

Implant information

Serial #   _____
Lot #   _____
Catalog #   _____
Size   _____

Name of plastic surgeon   _____
Date of surgery   _____
Location of Surgery   _____
Were biopsies performed? Yes or No
If yes, be sure to retain a copy of your pathology report

Also be sure to obtain a copy of your operative report.

DATE AND TIMES OF FOLLOW-UP APPOINTMENTS

Month	Day	Time
_____	_____	_____
_____	_____	_____
_____	_____	_____
_____	_____	_____
_____	_____	_____

NOTES

LIPOSUCTION WORKSHEET

Before surgery, it is important to understand the technique that will be used for your liposuction procedure. While some patients may be hesitant to discuss things in detail, it is very important to understand exactly what will and won't happen during your surgery.

What technique will be used?

Tumescent technique
Other _____

Will your liposuction procedure be power assisted?

Yes _____ No _____

Check which specific technique the plastic surgeon will be performing.

Specific Technique: _____
Ultrasonic _____
Other _____

How many liters of tumescent fluid will be removed?

_____

Expect it to be infiltrated. Write this number down. Anything over five liters is considered high volume and may increase risk of complications.

Where will the incisions be made?

Have these marked by the plastic
surgeon in your consultation
prior to your surgery date.

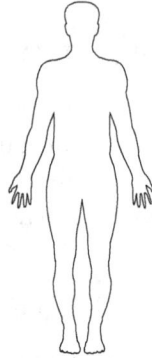

**Where will the surgery be performed? Is it in the office, at an
ambulatory surgical center, or at the hospital?**

_____

Is the facility licensed? _____
Is it Medicare approved? _____
Is it state certified? _____

**Does the surgeon use the services of a nurse anesthetist or an
anesthesiologist that is a diplomat of the American Board of
Anesthesiology? This is very important; there is a difference.**

_____

_____

What is the anesthesiologist's name? _____
Number of years in practice? _____
Malpractice record? _____

Have all consent forms been reviewed? Questions should be discussed with the plastic surgeon.

Yes _____ No _____

Examination of the specific areas to be liposuctioned with the plastic surgeon. Twice is preferred, allowing both the patient and surgeon to see any irregularities of the skin, including contour deformities, depressions, and scars from previous surgeries.

Do you have the required postoperative garments?

Abdominal binder, girdles, etc.?
Ask where to buy these or if they will be provided by the plastic surgeon.

Postoperative visits. Write down the dates and times of your postoperative days, including the day of suture removal.

DATE AND TIMES OF FOLLOW-UP APPOINTMENTS

Month	Day	Time
_____	_____	_____
_____	_____	_____
_____	_____	_____
_____	_____	_____
_____	_____	_____

Have you reviewed your postoperative instructions? These should be reviewed with the doctor and consultant. Make sure that all of your questions are thoroughly answered.

NOTES

Glossary

A

abdominoplasty (tummy tuck) – a procedure that minimizes the abdominal area. In abdominoplasty, the surgeon makes a long incision from one side of the hipbone to the other. Excess fat and skin are surgically removed from the middle and lower abdomen and the muscles of the abdomen wall are tightened.

Accreditation Association for Ambulatory Surgical Facilities (AAASF) – See "Quad A."

aesthetic plastic surgery (cosmetic plastic surgery) – one type of plastic surgery performed to repair or reshape otherwise normal structures of the body, primarily to improve the patient's appearance and self-esteem.

anchor scar technique (Wise-pattern technique) – the most common and conventional method of performing a surgical breast reduction that leaves a characteristic "anchor scar" on the underside of the breast.

anesthesia – lack of a normal sensation brought on by an anesthetic drug.

areola – dark area of skin that surrounds the nipple of the breast.

aspirator – suction device; used in liposuction.

asymmetry – lacking symmetry; parts of the body are unequal in shape or size compared with their opposites, e.g., one breast larger than the other.

augmentation mammaplasty (breast augmentation) – a procedure to reshape the breast in order to make it larger. The procedure can also be performed to reconstruct the breast following breast surgery.

B

bariatric body contouring – weight reduction treatment that surgically reduces the size of the stomach organ.

belt lipectomy – surgical removal of excess fat from around the entire circumference of the trunk instead of just the front (as with abdominoplasty).

board certified – in general, the formal statement that a physician has met the basic requirements, in education, training, experience and results, to practice a certain medical specialty, such as plastic surgery. You should find a doctor who is recognized by the American Board of Medical Specialties and is a diplomat or is certified by the American Board of Plastic Surgery (ABPS).

botox – short for "botulinum toxin" used by plastic surgeons to smooth wrinkles in the glabellar region.

breast aplasia (amastia) – rare condition in which the normal growth of the breast or nipple never takes place. They are congenitally absent. There is no sign whasotever of the breast tissue, nipple or areola.

breast augmentation (augmentation mammaplasty) – a procedure to reshape the breast in order to make it larger. The procedure can also be performed to reconstruct the breast following breast surgery.

breast dysphoria – acute dissatisfaction and unhappiness with the appearance of the breasts where there is normal function

breast hypoplasia – underdevelopment of the breast caused by insufficient mammary (milk-producing) tissue. Can also involve breast asymmetry.

breast lift (mastopexy) – the surgical raising and reshaping of sagging breasts (for a time). Can also reduce the size of the areola – the darker skin surrounding the nipple. If a woman's breasts are small or have lost volume, e.g., after pregnancy, breast implants inserted in conjunction with mastopexy can increase both the size and firmness of the breasts.

breast reduction – the opposite of breast augmentation; the size of the breast is reduced by surgically removing some of the underlying tissue.

C

cannula – hollow tube, usually plastic, with many medical applications, including liposuction.

capsular contracture – the most common complication of breast reconstruction surgery. Capsules of tightly-woven collagen fibers form as an immune response around a foreign body (eg. breast implants, pacemakers, orthopedic joint prosthetics), tending to wall it off. Capsular contracture occurs if the scar, or "capsule," around the implant begins to tighten. Can be very painful and can distort the appearance of the implant.

capsulectomy – surgical procedure to remove a post-surgical "capsule" such as the kind that forms around breast implants.

capsulorrhaphy – surgical procedure to correct "bottoming out" of a breast implant by tightening the internal capsule.

capsulotomy – surgical procedure to release a post-surgical "capsule" such as the kind that forms around breast implants.

Computed Axial Tomography scan (CAT scan or just CT scan) – a diagnostic imaging procedure that uses a combination of x-rays and computer technology to produce cross-sectional images (often called slices), both horizontally and vertically, of the body. A CT scan shows detailed images of any part of the body, including the bones, muscles, fat, and organs. CT scans are more detailed than general x-rays.

congenital – present at birth.

cosmetic plastic surgery (aesthetic plastic surgery) – one type of plastic surgery performed to repair or reshape otherwise normal structures of the body, primarily to improve the patient's appearance and self-esteem.

D

dermabrasion – a procedure that removes fine wrinkles and/or minimizes scars on the skin; involves the surgeon utilizing a high-speed rotating brush to remove the top layer of skin. The size and depth of the scars, as well as the degree of wrinkling, determine the appropriate level of skin that will be surgically sloughed.

dermis – the thick, sensitive layer of skin or connective tissue beneath the epidermis that contains blood, lymph vessels, sweat glands and nerve endings

displacement technique mammography – method of performing mammograms in women with breast implants. Requires the implant, either silicone gel or saline, to have been placed partly below and partly above the pectoral muscle.

E

epidermis – the thin, outermost layer of the skin; made up of several layers, it protects the underlying dermis.

expander/implant breast reconstruction – the use of an expander to create a breast mound, followed by the placement with a permanently filled breast implant.

extrusion – when the breast implant comes through the skin; unstable or weakened tissue covering and/or interruption of wound healing may result in extrusion.

G

gastric bypass – extreme treatment for morbid obesity in which the size of the stomach is surgically reduced.

gigantomastia (bilateral breast hypertrophy) – overly large breasts for a woman's proportion, often requiring breast reduction surgery to restore a natural appearance.

gynecomastia – a condition in which the male's breast tissue enlarges. Gynecomastia literally means "woman breast." This increase in tissue usually occurs at times when the male is having hormonal changes, such as during infancy, adolescence, and old age.

H

hemangioma (strawberry nevus) – an abnormal buildup of blood vessels in the skin or internal organs. The classic hemangioma appears as a red skin lesion that may be in the top layers (capillary hemangioma) or deeper in the skin (cavernous hemangioma) or both.

hematoma – an accumulation of blood that collects under the skin or in an organ, generally as the result of hemorrhage. Hematomas exist as bruises (ecchymoses) and can gradually migrate as the effused cells and pigment move into the connective tissue.

hypertrophic scarring – scarring in which the collagen produced to fill in a wound in the skin does not exceed the boundaries of the original wound.

hypotrophic scarring – scarring which are sunken and often hyperpigmented appearance due to a loss of collagen and ground substance, can also be problematic. Acne and chicken pox are two common conditions that frequently result in hypotrophic scarring. Stretch marks, which usually develop during pregnancy or adolescence due to rapid expansion of the skin, are another form of hypotrophic scar.

I

inframammary fold – fold at the bottom of the breast where it meets the skin of the chest.

intersternal distance – the distance between breast folds. This is a key measurement to determine how much cleavage a woman can expect from plastic surgery.

intraperitoneal – within the abdominal cavity. Fat in this location cannot be removed surgically.

K

keloid scarring – scarring in which raised, reddish nodules appear at the site of a wound in the skin, often extending beyond the boundaries of the original wound. Most common in people with darker skin tones.

L

Liposuction (lipoplasty, also known as "liposculpture," "suction lipectomy" and "suction-assisted lipectomy") – a procedure that removes excess fat from under the skin through a suctioning process. Although liposuction is not a substitute for weight loss, it is a way of changing the body's shape and contour through the removal of excess fat tissue.

M

mammogram – X-ray examination of the breast

mastectomy – surgery to remove portions of or all of the breast

mastopexy (full breast lift) – surgical procedure to repair the most severe breast sagging, ptosis grade III. This procedure will also result in an "anchor scar."

migration – movement of gel from an implant to the lymph nodes under the arm, and possible to other locations in the body, after a silicone implant ruptures.

Mondor's cords – Firm, cord-like bands that sometimes form just under the skin near the breast. They are temporary but often painful. Most commonly caused by an incision on or near the breast.

N

necrosis – the death of living tissue

nipple aplasia – see "breast aplasia."

nipple hypoplasia – see "breast hypoplasia."

P

panniculectomy – the surgical removal of excess abdominal panniculus, called the "apron" in layman's terms, which is that redundant layer of fat tissue at the lowest portion of the abdominal wall.

partial abdominoplasty – a "mini tummy tuck." This procedure is ideal for individuals who have fat deposits limited to the area below the navel.

partial subcutaneous mastectomy – direct extraction of glandular and fatty tissue from the region directly behind the areola through an incision under the nipple.

pectoralis major muscle – the thick, fan-shaped muscle situated at the upper front (anterior) of the chest wall which makes up the bulk of the chest muscles in the male and which lies under the breast in the female.

periareolar approach – surgery on the breast performed through an incision under the areola.

periareolar lift (crescent lift) – surgical procedure in which a small amount of skin is removed from above the areola permitting repositioning of the nipple complex to improve the appearance of mildly sagging breasts.

plastic surgery – the surgical specialty that deals with the reconstruction of facial and body tissue that requires a reshaping or remolding due to disease, a defect, or disorder - in order to approximate a normal appearance (cosmetic plastic surgery) or to restore function (reconstructive plastic surgery).

Poland syndrome – a chest wall anomaly usually involving ipsilateral breast and nipple hypoplasia and/or aplasia, deficiency of subcutaneous fat and axillary hair, absence of the sternal head of the pectoralis major, hypoplasia of the rib cage and hypoplasia of the upper extremity.

ptosis – degree of sag in the breasts, determined by the position of the nipple with respect to the inframammary fold.

Q

Quad A – the Accreditation Association for Ambulatory Surgical Facilities (AAASF) which verifies that a surgical facility meets and maintains national standards for surgical environments. Their ratings indicate the level of anaesthesia they are permitted to administer, which is an accurate indicator of the degree of difficulty they are prepared to treat.

R

reconstructive plastic surgery – one type of plastic surgery that is performed on abnormal structures of the body that may be caused by trauma, infection, developmental abnormalities, congenital defects, disease, or tumors. This type of surgery is usually performed to improve function but may also be performed to approximate a normal appearance.

revision surgery – a follow-on operation at the site of a previous surgery to correct problems of capsular contracture, wrinkling, asymmetry, rupture/ deflation, extrusion, implant malposition or other local complications.

S

saline breast implant – one of two types of breast implants, the other being silicone gel. Saline is preferred by many women because it is made of a natural ingredient – salt water.

scar – a scar is the mark left on the skin after the healing of a cut, burn or other wound. Collagen forms to fill in the wound or incision. Scarring is the body's natural way of healing and replacing lost or damaged skin. See "hypertrophic" and "keloid" scarring. Although scarring is a common complication of surgery, the 6-7% rate reported for augmentation patients by the two main manufacturers in the world, Allergan and Mentor, is a notable complication for a cosmetic procedure.

seroma – a pocket of clear "serous" fluid that sometimes develops in the body after surgery. When small blood vessels are ruptured blood plasma, or sera, can seep out. Inflammation caused by dying cells also contributes to the fluid. Seromas are different from hematomas (which contain red blood cells) and abscesses (which contain pus and result from infection).

severe congenital breast deformity – a birth defect which results in one or both breasts being entirely missing, grossly underformed, or grossly asymmetrically formed

silicone gel breast implant – one of two types of breast implants, the other being saline, commonly used to enlarge and re-shape the breast. Some patients have reported post-operative problems with silicone gel implants which include connective tissue disorders and other illnesses, but no causal link has been established to date.

subcutaneous fat deficiency – inadequate or underdeveloped fat deposits under the skin.

subcuticular closure – sutures placed under the skin. This technique helps to reduce scarring.

subpectoral (dual plane) technique – a method of surgically implanting breast enlargements by placing one-half to two-thirds of the implant under the pectoral muscle and the remainder above the pectoral muscle. Gives a more natural appearance than putting the whole implant either over or under the pectoral muscle, but it takes more skill to accomplish.

symmastia (also known as breadloafing, kissing implants, and "uniboob") – a condition in which breast implants merge in the middle of the chest. Often caused by over-disection of the tissues in the cleavage area. More prevalent among thin women and those suffering from pectus excavatum (depressed breastbone).

T

transaxillary approach – method of implanting a breast augmentation through an incision made under the arm

TUBA (transumbilical) – any surgical procedure performed via entry through the umbilicus (belly button).

tubular breast deformities – breast condition usually involving herniation of breast tissue into the nipple areola region and/or inadequate development of the inferior half of the breast, affecting both the size and shape of the breast.

tumescent liposuction technique – a method of performing liposuction in which the area to be suctioned is first infiltrated with fluids.

tummy tuck (abdominoplasty) – a procedure that minimizes the abdominal area. In abdominoplasty, the surgeon makes a long incision from one side of the hipbone to the other. Excess fat and skin are surgically removed from the middle and lower abdomen and the muscles of the abdomen wall are tightened.

V

vertical lift – surgical procedure to improve the appearance of moderately sagging breasts by removing a "donut" of skin around the areolar complex and lifting the portion under the areola in the vertical dimension.

ABOUT THE AUTHOR

Dr. Stuart Linder, M.D., F.A.C.S.

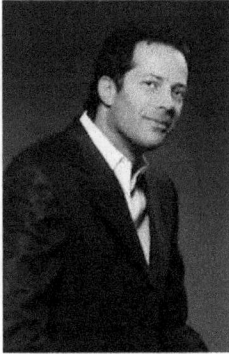

Dr. Stuart Linder is a board certified plastic and reconstructive surgeon based in Beverly Hills, California. He specializes in breast augmentation, breast reduction and body sculpting. Dr. Linder has received a degree in Biology and Psychology and a Medical Degree from the University of California, Los Angeles. In 1994, Dr. Linder went on to receive his general surgery residency at UCLA Medical Center and later his Plastic Surgery Fellowship.

Dr. Linder is affiliated with numerous organizations including the American Board of Plastic Surgery, the American College of Surgeons and the American Society of Plastic & Reconstructive Surgeons.

Dr. Linder has appeared on numerous television shows discussing plastic surgery including MTV, E! Entertainment, The Learning Channel, Discovery Health, "Women to Women" and "The Other Half." In addition to his national appearances, Dr Linder has provided insight and expertise to local networks and independent stations. Media representatives will often contact Dr. Linder on breaking news stories related to breast augmentation and reduction as well as liposuction and the latest technology. He has also been featured in several magazines and journals as well as appeared on numerous radios talk shows and radio news bureaus.

Dr. Linder resides in Beverly Hills with his wife and two children.

www.ingramcontent.com/pod-product-compliance
Lightning Source LLC
Chambersburg PA
CBHW062221270326
41930CB00009B/1812